Contents

CW01499622

Acknowledgements

This Trainer has been developed by Cambridge University Press and Assessment using experienced material writers and trainers, in collaboration with OET and with Cambridge English Language Assessment reviewers and SMEs (Specialist Medical Experts).

We would like to thank Nick Kenny (writer/audio recording coordinator/reviewer), Catherine Leyshon (writer), David Clark (writer), Susan White (writer), Jessica Worthing (writer), Gurleen Khaira (writer), Eleanor Lindberg (writer), Shakina Mohol (writer), Judith Wilson (reviewer), Joanna Kosta (reviewer), Susan Kingsley (reviewer), Nicola Mooney (reviewer), Liz Shrubsall (reviewer), Angela McCarthy (reviewer), Dr Paul Siklos (SME), Dr Alexander Leguia (SME) and Jane Broadley (SME) for their work on the material.

The writers and publishers acknowledge the following sources of copyright material and are grateful for the permissions granted. While every effort has been made, it has not always been possible to identify the sources of all the material used, or to trace all copyright holders. If any omissions are brought to our notice, we will be happy to include the appropriate acknowledgements on reprinting and in the next update to the digital edition, as applicable.

Please note that the medical texts used for the development of the practice tests, particularly those covering medical practice, policy, guidelines and procedures, are based on published information available at the time of writing. There will be variations in practice from one medical institution to the next, and many documents will be subject to change. Neither Cambridge University Press and Assessment nor the rights holders are responsible for any discrepancies between the information contained here and current medical policy.

Keys: Test = T, Part = P

Text

Reading:

T1PB: Drug Safety Update date volume 7 issue 4, November 2013: A1 licensed under the Open Government Licence v3.0; **T1PC:** BMJ Publishing Group Limited for the text taken from 'Arun Bhaskar: The inescapable truth: palliative care is not enough—we can and should legislate for assisted dying'. Copyright © 2022 BMJ Publishing Group Limited. All rights reserved. Reproduced with permission; New Scientist for the adapted text 'The surprising, ancient origins of TB, humanity's most deadly disease' by Rebecca Batley. Copyright ©2021 New Scientist Ltd. All rights reserved. Distributed by Tribune Content Agency; **T2PB:** RCVS for the text taken from 'Euthanasia of animals'. Copyright © 2021 Royal College of Veterinary Surgeons. Reproduced with kind permission; **T2PC:** The Scientist for the text taken from 'Return of the Worms' by Catherine Offord. Copyright © 2021 The Scientist now part of the LabX Media Group. Reproduced by permission of The Scientist; **T3PC:** Guardian News & Media Ltd for the text taken from 'Fibromyalgia may be a condition of the immune system not the brain – study' by Linda Geddes. Copyright © 2022 Guardian News & Media Ltd. Reproduced with permission; **T4PA:** Egton Medical Information Systems Limited for the text taken from 'Blepharitis' by Dr Laurence Knott. Copyright © 2021 Egton Medical Information Systems Limited. All rights reserved. Reproduced under licence from www.Patient.info; **T6PA:** Egton Medical Information Systems Limited for the text taken from 'Pyelonephritis' by Mary Harding. Copyright © 2016 Egton Medical Information Systems Limited. All rights reserved. Reproduced under licence from www.Patient.info; **T4PB:** Nottingham University Hospitals NHS Trust for the text taken from 'Decontamination of Reusable Invasive Medical Devices Policy including Risks Related to Creutzfeldt - Jakob Disease (CJD)' by Carl Yates. Copyright © 2020 Nottingham University Hospitals NHS Trust. All rights reserved; Nottingham University Hospitals NHS Trust for the text taken from 'Isolation Policy' by Infection Prevention and Control Team. Copyright © 2022 Nottingham University Hospitals NHS Trust. All rights reserved; **T4PC:** Taylor & Francis for the text taken from The treatment of phantom limb pain using immersive virtual reality: Three case studies by Craig D. Murray, Stephen Pettifer, et al. Copyright © 2007 Taylor & Francis. Permission conveyed through Copyright Clearance Center, Inc; Guardian News & Media Ltd for the text taken from 'Depression is not a one-size-fits-all condition – we need a more nuanced approach to mental health' by Sidney Bloch. Copyright © 2022 Guardian News & Media Ltd. Reproduced by permission; **T5PA:** Clarity Informatics Limited for the text taken from 'Shingles: How should I diagnose shingles?'. Copyright © 2021 The NICE Clinical Knowledge Summaries (CKS). Reproduced by permission of Clarity Informatics Limited; Clarity Informatics Limited for the text taken from 'Antiviral treatment'. Copyright © The NICE Clinical Knowledge Summaries (CKS). Reproduced by permission of Clarity Informatics Limited; Clarity Informatics Limited for the text taken from 'Antiviral drugs'. Copyright © 2021 The NICE Clinical Knowledge Summaries (CKS). Reproduced by permission of Clarity Informatics Limited; Clarity Informatics Limited for the text taken from 'Complications'. Copyright © 2021 The NICE Clinical Knowledge Summaries (CKS). Reproduced by permission of Clarity Informatics Limited; Clarity Informatics Limited or the text taken from

'Pain-management'. Copyright © 2021 The NICE Clinical Knowledge Summaries (CKS). Reproduced by permission of Clarity Informatics Limited; **T5PB:** Text taken from 'Updated NACI recommendation for measles post-exposure prophylaxis' by The Public Health Agency of Canada licensed under the Open Government Licence – Canada; Nottingham University Hospitals NHS Trust for the text taken from 'Guideline for allowing children to visit patients on the Adult Critical Care Unit' by Ruth Pettit, Sister Adult Critical Care. Copyright © 2019 Nottingham University Hospitals NHS Trust. All rights reserved; Text taken from 'Guidelines for the Infection Control Management of Inpatients with Tuberculosis' by Vickie Longstaff, Homerton University Hospital, NHS foundation trust licensed under the Open Government Licence; Text taken from 'Policy and Procedure for the Safe and Effective Use of Bed Safety Sides for Adult and Paediatric Patients', Homerton University Hospital, NHS foundation trust licensed under the Open Government Licence; **T5PC:** BMJ Publishing Group Ltd. & The Health Foundation for the text taken from 'Sleep deprivation and starvation in hospitalised patients: how medical care can harm patients' by Tim Xu, Elizabeth C Wick, Martin A Makary. Copyright © 2016, BMJ Publishing Group Ltd. & The Health Foundation. Permission conveyed through Copyright Clearance Center, Inc; BMJ Publishing Group Ltd. & The Health Foundation for the text taken from 'Heading, concussion, and dementia: how medicine is changing football forever' by Luke Taylor. Copyright © 2021, BMJ Publishing Group Ltd. Permission conveyed through Copyright Clearance Center, Inc; **T6PA:** Egton Medical Information Systems Limited for the text taken from 'Pyelonephritis' by Dr Laurence Knott. Copyright © 2022 Egton Medical Information Systems Limited. All rights reserved. Reproduced under licence from www.Patient.info; **T6PB:** NHS Tayside for the text taken from 'NHS Tayside Policy: Safe use of Entonox for short term pain relief' by Alan Stirling. Copyright © 2022 NHS Tayside. Reproduced with kind permission; NHS Tayside for the text taken from 'NHS Tayside Policy: Just in Case Boxes in Primary Care' by Shirley Kelly. Copyright © 2021 NHS Tayside. Reproduced with kind permission of Shirley Kelly; NHS Tayside for the text taken from 'Summoning Clinical Assistance' by Dr Peter Currie. Copyright © 2021 NHS Tayside. Reproduced with kind permission of Morag MacRae on behalf of the Summoning Clinical Assistance and Adult Missing Patient policy authors; **T6PC:** ABC for the text taken from 'Can 'lifestyle medicine' such as diet, exercise and mindfulness help treat chronic pain?' by Kate Midena. Copyright © 2021 ABC. Reproduced by permission of the Australian Broadcasting Corporation; The President and Fellows of Harvard College for the text taken from 'Predicting Side Effects' by Stephanie Dutchen. Copyright © 2020 The President and Fellows of Harvard College. Reproduced by kind permission.

Listening:

T1PC: EMAP Publishing Limited the text taken from 'Giving patients a voice will help shift outdated perceptions of mental health hospitals' by John-Barry Waldron. Copyright © 2019 EMAP Publishing Limited. Reproduced with permission; EMAP Publishing Limited the text taken from 'Bringing care closer to home for people with idiopathic pulmonary fibrosis. Copyright © 2019 EMAP Publishing Limited. Reproduced with permission; **T2PC:** EMAP Publishing Limited for the text taken from 'Evaluating a children's learning resource to improve handwashing behavior'. Copyright © 2021 EMAP Publishing Limited. Reproduced with kind permission; **T4PB:** EMAP Publishing Limited for the text taken from 'Preventing facial skin damage beneath personal protective equipment'. Copyright © 2020 EMAP Publishing Limited. Reproduced with permission; **T5PB:** EMAP Publishing Limited for the text taken from 'Early mobilisation 3: moving patients from their bed to chair without aids'. Copyright © 2021 EMAP Publishing Limited. Reproduced with permission; **T5PC:** EMAP Publishing Limited for the text taken from 'The benefits and drawbacks of open and restricted visiting hours'. Copyright © 2018 EMAP Publishing Limited. Reproduced with permission; EMAP Publishing Limited for the text taken from 'The principles of maggot therapy and its role in contemporary wound care'. Copyright © 2021 EMAP Publishing Limited. Reproduced with permission; **T6PC:** BMJ Publishing Group Ltd. & British Thoracic Society for the text taken from 'Improving the global diagnosis and management of asthma in children' by Warren Lenney, Andrew Bush, Dominic A Fitzgerald, Monica Fletcher, Anders Ostrem, Soren Pedersen, Stanley J Szefler, Heather J Zar. Copyright © 2018 BMJ Publishing Group Ltd. & British Thoracic Society. Permission conveyed through Copyright Clearance Center, Inc.

Photography

Cover photography by Tom Merton/OJO Images/Getty Images and The Good Brigade/DigitalVision/Getty Images.

Audio

Audio produced and recorded at dSound, London

Typesetting

Designed and typeset by QBS Learning

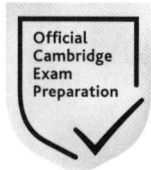

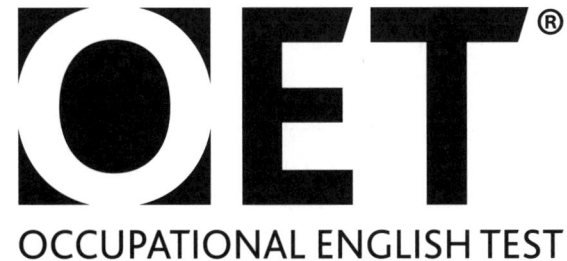

OCCUPATIONAL ENGLISH TEST

Trainer

Medicine

Six Practice Tests

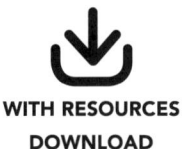

WITH RESOURCES
DOWNLOAD

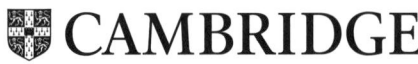

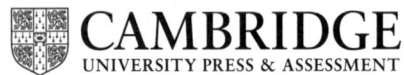

Shaftesbury Road, Cambridge CB2 8EA, United Kingdom

One Liberty Plaza, 20th Floor, New York, NY 10006, USA

477 Williamstown Road, Port Melbourne, VIC 3207, Australia

314–321, 3rd Floor, Plot 3, Splendor Forum, Jasola District Centre, New Delhi – 110025, India

103 Penang Road, #05–06/07, Visioncrest Commercial, Singapore 238467

Cambridge University Press & Assessment is a department of the University of Cambridge.

We share the University's mission to contribute to society through the pursuit of education, learning and research at the highest international levels of excellence.

www.cambridge.org
Information on this title: www.cambridge.org/9781009162920

First published 2023

20 19 18 17 16 15 14 13 12 11 10 9 8 7 6 5 4 3 2 1

Printed in Dubai by Oriental Press

A catalogue record for this publication is available from the British Library

ISBN 978-1-009-16292-0 OET Trainer for Medicine with answers with audio

Additional resources for this publication at www.cambridge.org/go

Cambridge University Press & Assessment has no responsibility for the persistence or accuracy of URLs for external or third-party internet websites referred to in this publication and does not guarantee that any content on such websites is, or will remain, accurate or appropriate.

Introduction

Who is *OET Trainer* for?

This book is suitable for anyone who is preparing to take the OET (Occupational English Test) for healthcare professionals. OET is recognised by healthcare trusts, boards and councils in the UK, the USA, Australia, Ireland, New Zealand, Singapore and Dubai amongst others as proof of a candidate's ability to communicate effectively in a healthcare environment and covers a number of medical professions. This book focuses on the medical speciality of Medicine. It is designed both for self-study or to be used by teachers for preparing students for the exam. All users can access or download a variety of support materials via an access code on the inside front cover for our Cambridge One online platform, such as answer keys, audio files and transcripts, and an eBook, and with audios also available via QR codes accessible on your smartphone, so that you can even study on the go.

What is *OET Trainer*?

OET Trainer for Medicine contains six authentic practice tests for the exam, covering the four papers, or sub-tests, that form the complete exam: Reading, Listening, Speaking and Writing. The first two tests in the Trainer are 'guided tests', which means they include extra training and information to familiarise you with each part of the exam, what it tests and the skills and kinds of language that can help you to complete the exam tasks successfully. Tests 3 to 6 are purely practice tests. All six tests match the exam in format and standard.

In Test 1, each part of each of the papers/sub-tests is introduced separately in the form of a **Training** section and an **Exam Practice** section. The **Training** sections give key information about each part of the exam in the **Task Information**, and have advice and guidance to help you understand what each task is testing, alongside exercises that will build the language and skills directly relevant to each.

An **Exam Practice** section follow each **Training** section. Authentic versions of each task are accompanied by an **Action Plan**, which gives step-by-step guidance on how to approach the task, alongside tips on general exam strategy. For the Reading and Listening exam tasks, there is also **Advice** linked to specific questions, providing hints and clues to guide you through your first exposure to the tasks.

Test 2 follows a similar pattern to Test 1 in that it also consists of **Training** and **Exam Practice** sections to review and further develop important skills, language and exam task familiarity. The **Exam Practice** section follows the same format as Test 1, with the exception of the **Action Plan**, which is simply referenced.

Test 3 to 6 are complete practice tests without advice or training. They give you the opportunity to put into practice the skills, language and strategies you have acquired while working through Tests 1 and 2.

All tests have an **Explanatory Answer Key** (see next section).

Features of *OET Trainer*

- An **Explanatory Answer Key** is available for download via the Cambridge One online platform. It is 'explanatory' in the sense that it not only provides you with the correct answers for the tests, but also where relevant, explains why the answers are correct and why other options are not.

- For Writing tasks, the **Explanatory Answer Key** provides **model answers** for you to compare your answers with, with notes on how the model was put together.

- A **Listening transcript** is also provided via Cambridge One for all audio tracks in the Training as well as for the Listening exam tasks themselves.

- Full **Downloadable Audio** is available for all tracks, covering both the Listening exam tasks and Listening and Speaking Training sections. In addition, each audio track has a QR code alongside the activity, permitting you to access individual tracks via your smartphone, allowing you to practice Listening activities wherever you are. Note that if your smartphone does not come with a QR code reader, you will need to download a third-party QR reader app to use this feature.

- An **Interactive eBook version** of the print book is also available via the code in the print book, allowing online access via our Cambridge One platform. All audio tracks are included in the eBook.

- **Marking criteria** for the Speaking and Writing papers (sub-tests) are provided at the end of the print book to help you understand what you are being assessed on in these two sub-tests, and where relevant, are referenced by the Training sections, so that you can see how Training exercises are focussed on helping you score well in each criterion.

How to use the *OET Trainer*

Test 1 Training

- For each part of each paper (sub-test), you should begin by studying the **Task Information**, which provides an overview of each part and, depending on the task, covers key information, such as the task description, task style, duration and timings, rules to observed during the exam and even the skills and language that will aid in its completion.

- Throughout Test 1 Training, you will also information marked **Tip!** These tips relate to both specific aspects of the Training and more generic practical information to help you understand complete the tasks you will face in the actual exam.

- The exercises in the Training cover skills and language that will help you deal with all the practice tests in this book as well as the actual test itself.

- The answers to all the training exercises are included in the **Explanatory Answer Key**, and just like the answers for the practice tests themselves, are, where required, detailed to the extent that they not only provide the correct answers, but also explanations as to why other answers or approaches are incorrect.

Test 1 Exam Practice

- Start by looking at the **Action Plan**, which gives you a set of recommendations of how best to deal with each exam part or task on the day of the exam itself. Depending on the task/part, you may even get pointers on what to do BEFORE, DURING or AFTER the task.

- Then look at the practice exam task itself. For receptive skill tasks (Reading and Listening) you will find **Advice** sections, which provide hints on what to look/listen for in each question in the task. For productive skills (Writing and Speaking), there are more **Tips!** which point out aspects of the specific task you should be aware of. Such **Tips!** will commonly refer to points covered in the preceding Training sections as well as covering general FAQs (Frequently Asked Questions) that candidates have about the exam.

- As ever, the downloadable **Explanatory Answer Key** will provide not only correct answers, but also explanations as to why they are correct and other options are not, or a model text in the case of the Writing paper (sub-test). Note that for obvious reasons, a model answer is not provided for the Speaking paper. However, Speaking tests do include the examiner's role cards so you can use them to understand/predict the general structure of each role play.

Test 2 Training and Exam Practice

- The Test 2 Training and Exam Practice build on, develop, extend and review what has been covered in Test 1.
- The same features are present such as **Tip!** and **Advice** to guide you through the new exam task being practised, but note that some sections such as **Task Information** and **Action Plan** are not repeated.

Tests 3 to 6 Exam Practice

- In Tests 3, 4, 5 and 6 you should apply the skills, techniques, strategies, and language you have practised in Tests 1 and 2.
- You can do these tests and the papers within them in any order, but you are encouraged to stick to the time recommendations, in order to better recreate exam conditions when practising.
- Note that for OET Listening papers, unlike like many Cambridge exams, you will only hear the audios one time.
- It will be easier to keep to the exam instructions and recreate exam conditions if can find somewhere quiet to work, and if you give yourself enough time to do each paper in its entirety. That said, it is perfectly feasible to take a bite-size approach and break down the papers into individual tasks. Remember that each part of the Listening paper has its own separate audio, accessible via QR code on your smartphone, so you can practise whilst on the go.
- As mentioned, the Speaking paper comes with the role card for both candidate and examiner. Ideally, you would work with another candidate or health specialist to practise the Speaking paper. If working on your own, you can see the examiner's role card, which will help you understand what you might be expected to say during your 'turns'.

Overview of OET exam papers (sub-tests)

Reading 60 minutes

The Reading sub-test consists of three parts and has a total of 42 question items. All three parts take in total 60 minutes to complete. The topics are of generic healthcare interest and are therefore accessible to candidates across all professions.

Part A comes separately from Parts B and C and has two parts: a text booklet with the four texts you have to read and a separate question paper. You have 15 minutes for this part and then your answers will be collected. Part A is an expeditious reading task and has three sets of questions. The first part is always a multiple matching exercise. The second two parts are short answer questions and sentence completion questions. Note that the number of each of these types of questions may vary from test to test, but in total there will be 13 questions.

Parts B and C comes together in one paper, and include both texts and the questions papers. The focus in both parts is on careful reading. You have 45 minutes in total to complete these two parts.

Part	Task Types	No. of questions	Format	Task Information
A	Multiple matching	7 (may vary)	Four short texts on the same healthcare topic. Candidates' ability to quickly and efficiently locate specific information is tested, with candidates asked either to identify which of the texts contains information or to find specific information within the texts.	Page 10
	Short answer questions / Sentence completion	13 (may vary)		
B	Multiple choice	6	Six short healthcare workplace texts (100–150 words). Each text has a single three-option multiple choice question.	Page 18
C	Multiple choice	16	Two longer texts (800 words) on topics of interest to healthcare professionals with eight four-option multiple choice questions on each.	Page 24

Writing 45 minutes

The Writing sub-test takes 45 minutes and is profession-specific. There is one task set for each profession based on a typical workplace situation and the demands of the profession – a nurse does the task for nursing, a dentist does the task for dentistry, and so on.

The Writing paper is assessed against six criteria. For more details of these criteria, please refer to page 212.

Task Type	No. of words	Format	Task Information
Letter	180–200	You write a letter, usually a referral letter, but possibly a letter of transfer or discharge, based on a set of information (case notes and/or other related documentation)	Page 35

Listening approximately 40 minutes

The OET Listening sub-test consists of three parts, and a total of 42 question items. The topics are of generic healthcare interest and accessible to candidates across all professions. The total length of the Listening audio is about 40 minutes, including recorded speech and pauses to allow you time to write your answers. You will hear each recording once and are expected to write your answers while listening. In contrast to the Reading, all three parts of the Listening sub-test are in the same paper.

Part	Task Types	No. of questions	Format	Task Information
A	Sentence completion	24	You hear two extracts from medical consultations of about five minutes and need to complete a set of notes for each extract with a word or short phrase.	Page 40
B	Multiple choice	6	You hear six short extracts set in the healthcare workplace of about one minute in length. Each extract has a single three-option multiple choice question.	Page 45
C	Multiple choice	12	You hear two longer extracts on topics of interest to healthcare professionals in the form of an interview or presentation. Each is around five minutes in length and has six three-option multiple choice questions.	Page 50

Speaking approximately 20 minutes

The Speaking sub-test is delivered individually and takes around 20 minutes in total. This part of OET also uses materials specifically designed for your profession and is role play based. In each role play, you take your professional role (for example, as a nurse or as a pharmacist).

Note that before the role plays begin, there is a short warm-up conversation with the interlocutor about your professional background, which is not assessed. Note also that you have three minutes to prepare for each role play, during which time you can make notes on the role card and ask the interlocutor about anything you are unsure of.

The Speaking paper is assessed against various linguistic and clinical communication criteria. For more details of these criteria, please refer to page 214.

Task Type	Format	Task Information
Role play	You do two role plays of about five minutes in length. You are given role cards for each and the interlocutor has their own cards. For each role play, you deal with a typical workplace situation for your profession with the interlocutor typically playing the role of a patient, carer or parent.	Page 56

Further information

The information in this Trainer is designed to provide an overview of OET. For more detailed information on OET, including booking information, please visit the official OET website (www.occupationalenglishtest.org).

Task information

- Part A tests your ability to skim, scan and record information quickly and accurately.

- You read four short texts (A–D) typically encountered in the medical workplace on the same topic, usually a medical condition or procedure.

- Each text addresses a different aspect of the topic, and at least one text will be graphical, for example, a table, graph, or flow chart.

- The texts can contain a variety of information, such as dosages, how to administer medication, what advice to give patients, symptoms and risk factors.

- There are three sets of questions. The first set is a multiple matching task where you have to identify in which text certain pieces of information are located.

- The other two sets of questions (short answer questions and sentence completion) ask you to find specific information within the texts.

- For these sets of questions, each answer / piece of missing information is a precise word or short phrase in one of the texts.

- You have 15 minutes to answer 20 questions.

Skimming: identifying types of information in the four texts

Before you read the first set of questions, skim-read the texts to familiarise yourself with them so that you have a 'map' in your head of what type of information each contains.

1 Read the following statements about skim-reading and put a tick (✓) if they are correct and cross (✗) if they are incorrect.

   1 You use it to get an in-depth understanding of the text.

   2 You use it to get a general idea of the subject and purpose of a text.

   3 You use it to find specific words that you are looking for.

   4 You need to read the text slowly and carefully to ensure you understand every word.

   5 You focus on text features, such as format, structure, title, headings and sub-headings, graphical information, bold or highlighted information.

   6 For a paragraph or paragraphs of text, you move your eyes both horizontally and vertically across the text to find what you need.

Tip! You only have 15 minutes in total for Part A. Aim to skim all four texts in two minutes or less.

2 Look at Text A on the subject of inflammatory bowel disease on the opposite page. Quickly skim read the text (30 seconds). Think of a title or heading to describe its overall content.

Tip! Some Part A texts have clear titles which explain their overall content and some do not. Text B which we will see later has its own title.

Text A

Inflammatory bowel disease (IBD) is an umbrella term used to describe disorders that lead to chronic, relapsing intestinal inflammation. The two main types are:

Ulcerative colitis (UC): causes prolonged inflammation and sores (ulcers) in the colon and rectum

Crohn's disease (CD): characterised by inflammation of the digestive tract lining. Often extends deep into affected tissues.

Symptoms include: diarrhoea, fever, fatigue, abdominal pain and cramping, rectal bleeding, reduced appetite, unintended weight loss

Treatment aims to relieve and prevent recurrence of symptoms and includes:

Dietary and lifestyle changes:
- smaller and more frequent meals
- soft, bland foods & avoidance of trigger foods (fatty, fried, spicy, fibre-rich and dairy)
- stress management – relaxation therapies such as meditation
- adequate sleep & regular exercise

Medication:
- aminosalicylates or mesalazines
- immunosuppressants eg. steroids or azathioprine
- biologics
- antibiotics

Surgery: Approximately 25% of IBD patients will require surgery. Common reasons include poor reaction to medication or nutritional treatment, strictures in the intestine and abscesses or fistulas.

Text B

Classification of ulcerative colitis by severity

Symptoms	Severe	Mild
frequent defecation	> 6 times daily	< 4 times daily
fever	37.5 °C or higher	absent
tachycardia	90/min or more	absent
anaemia	Hb 10g/dl or less	absent
erythrocyte sedimentation rate (ESR)	30 mm/h or more	normal

3 Now look at the topic box below. Look at Text A again and also Text B which has a title. Skim read the texts to identify which of the topics are included in each.

Tip! Some topics may be mentioned in more than one text so you need to read the question carefully to understand which aspect of the topic you are looking for.

> medication types   dosages risk factors   types of treatment
> patient assessment administration   diagnosis   symptoms   definitions
> types of condition side-effects   investigations   (contra)indications
> patient advice   surgical

Text A topics: ....

Text B topics: ....

4 Look at the following Part A multiple-matching questions and focus on the underlined words. Match the words to the alternative ways they could be expressed. In which text can you find information about:

a) types or varieties

b) dietary and/or lifestyle changes

c) severity

Tip! The words used in the questions may be expressed differently in the four texts so think about the meaning of the questions rather than just focusing on the specific words in the questions.

1 how to assess the <u>seriousness</u> of an IBD?   ....

2 definitions of the different <u>kinds</u> of IBD?   ....

3 recommended <u>daily routine</u> <u>adjustments</u> for IBD patients.   ....

5 Look again at the questions in Exercise 4. Decide in which text (A or B) you are most likely to find the answer. Then scan-read the text to confirm your ideas.

Tip! There are usually seven of these multiple matching questions at the start of Part A.

Action plan

Remember that you only have 15 minutes for Part A, after which the Paper will be collected in. There are 20 questions and three question types with each requiring a slightly different approach. It is recommended that you try to answer the questions in order, as for example, doing the matching questions exercise first will help you for the later short answer and sentence completion questions.

Matching questions

1 Start by skim reading the texts to get an overview of the type of content each contains. Try not to spend more than a minute on each text.

2 Focus on text features, such as titles, headings, and words in bold that help you understand what information each text contains.

3 For each question, think about what is being asked for and decide which of the four texts you think most likely contains the information, based on your skim reading.

4 Check the text to confirm your ideas and if you cannot, check the next most probable text.

5 Indicate your answer by writing the capital letter of the text in the space provided.

Short answer and sentence completion questions

1 Read the questions / incomplete sentences and underline key words which help you decide what you are looking for and consider in which text you might find the answer.

2 Think about what type of information you are being asked for (a name, quantity, medication, etc.).

3 Scan the text you have chosen for the answer using the key words to guide you.

4 Write your answer (a word or short phrase) in the space provided clearly. Remember that the word or phrase required must be in the same form as it appears in the text.

5 For sentence completion questions, read through the sentence with the answer in place to check spelling, grammatical fit, that you haven't repeated words from the sentence and that the information is complete.

Pneumonia: Texts

Text A

Assessment, admission and discharge

The CURB65 score is used to determine 30-day mortality risk for patients with Community Acquired Pneumonia (CAP). It may also be used to inform admission and discharge decisions in conjunction with clinical judgement. Give 1 point for each of the following:

– Confusion: Abbreviated Mental Test Score <8
– blood Urea nitrogen: >7mmol/L
– Respiratory rate: >30 breaths / minute
– Blood pressure: systolic < 90 mmHg /diastolic < 60 mmHg
– age: >65

Admission guide:

>1: low risk → home care
>2: moderate risk → admission
>3 to 5: high risk → urgent admission / ICU care

Do not discharge patients with a score of 3 or above.

Before discharging, consider the following additional risk factors:

– temperature > 37.5°C
– heart rate >100 BPM
– oxygen saturation < 90% on room air
– inability to eat without assistance.

• End of life patients – agree approach for managing pneumonia in context of overall care plan.

• If a patient has a dementia diagnosis, the mental assessment must be adapted accordingly.

Text B

Information to give patients – community acquired pneumonia

Awareness of what to expect when recovering can help to reduce patients' anxiety and highlight the need to consult their healthcare professional if they feel that their condition is deteriorating or not improving as expected. Explain to patients that after starting treatment their symptoms should steadily improve, although the rate of improvement will vary with the severity of the pneumonia. It is expected that after:

1 week: fever resolved

4 weeks: chest pain and sputum production substantially reduced

6 weeks: cough and breathlessness substantially reduced

3 months: most symptoms resolved but fatigue may still be present

6 months: most people will feel back to normal

Provide patients with additional, specific advice regarding:

- possible adverse reactions to antibiotics.
- seeking medical help if symptoms worsen rapidly or significantly, if symptoms do not start to improve within three days, or if the person becomes systemically very unwell.

Text C

Thoracentesis procedure

A thoracentesis involves the removal of fluid from the pleural space. It involves the following steps.

1 Ask the patient to sit, leaning forwards, with their arms resting on a table.

2 Use auscultation and chest percussion to estimate the fluid height.

3 Select and mark the insertion point, one intercostal space below the top of the effusion. Insertion below the ninth rib should be avoided due to the risk of intra-abdominal injury. Prepare the insertion area and apply a sterile drape.

4 Use a 25-gauge needle to anaesthetise the skin over the insertion point.

5 Switch to a 22-gauge needle and advance this over the superior edge of the rib. In order to avoid intercostal vessel injury, the needle must not touch the inferior surface. Intermittently aspirate and inject.

6 Once pleural fluid is aspirated, withdraw slightly then inject additional anaesthetic to the highly sensitive parietal pleura. Note the penetration depth.

7 Attach an 18-gauge over-the-needle catheter to the syringe and advance over the superior aspect of the rib, pulling back while advancing. When fluid is aspirated, stop advancing, guide the catheter over the needle and remove the needle. Cover the open catheter hub to prevent air entering the pleural cavity.

8 Attach a syringe with a 3-way stopcock to the catheter hub. Aspirate the fluid required for diagnostic analysis (generally 50ml). If a larger amount is to be withdrawn for therapeutic reasons, attach a collection bag to the stopcock. Aspiration should be limited to 1500ml in order to avoid the risk of pleural edema or hypotension.

9 When aspiration is complete, ask the patient to hum whilst the catheter is removed. This lowers the chances of pneumothorax occurring. Cover the site with an occlusive dressing.

Complication	Comment	Treatment	
Bacteremia: Presence / multiplication of bacteria in the bloodstream	Untreated & clinically significant bacteremia progresses to SIRS, sepsis, septic shock and MODS.	Antibiotics (typically IV infusion)	
Acute Respiratory Distress Syndrome (ARDS) Build up of fluid in alveoli	More common in patients with severe pneumonia or chronic underlying lung diseases.	May require ventilation.	
Pleural effusion: Accumulation of fluid in pleura.			Antibiotics, drainage (thoracentesis, thoracostomy), pleurectomy.
Empyema: Infection of the fluid			
Pleurisy: Inflammation of pleura		NSAIDs	
Lung abscess: Formation of pus in a lung cavity.	Most frequently arises as a complication of aspiration pneumonia, caused by periodontal disease and poor oral hygiene.	Antibiotics. Surgical / percutaneous intervention required for abscesses > 6 cm. Lobectomy / pneumonectomy considered for patients who do not respond.	

Part A

TIME: 15 minutes

- Look at the four texts, **A–D**, in the separate **Text Booklet** that precedes the questions.
- For each question, **1–20**, look through the texts, **A–D**, to find the relevant information.
- Write your answers on the spaces provided in this **Question Paper**.
- Answer all the questions within the 15-minute time limit.
- Your answers should **only** be taken from texts **A–D** and must be correctly spelt.

Pneumonia: Questions

Questions 1–7

For each question, **1–7**, decide which text (**A**, **B**, **C** or **D**) the information comes from. You may use any letter more than once.

In which text can you find information about

1   the typical recovery timeline for pneumonia? _____

2   the definitions of medical terms related to pneumonia? _____

3   the equipment required to carry out a specific procedure. _____

4   patient guidance regarding medication side effects? _____

5   how to decide whether a patient should be hospitalised? _____

6   the underlying cause of some conditions associated with pneumonia? _____

7   the type of patient for whom the standard evaluation will need adapting? _____

> **Advice**
>
> **1** Look for information related to periods of time.
>
> **2** What punctuation sometimes introduces definitions?
>
> **3** The key word here is 'equipment'.
>
> **4** Which text's title tells you it refers to things to tell the patient?
>
> **5** Which text explains how to handle pneumonia patients?
>
> **6** Look for names of various conditions.
>
> **7** Which text explains how to handle pneumonia patients?

Questions 8–14

Answer each of the questions, **8–14**, with a word or short phrase from one of the texts. Each answer may include words, numbers or both.

8   Removing too much fluid during thoracentesis increases the risk of low blood pressure or _____ .

9   Most patients can expect to make a full recovery from pneumonia within _____ months.

10   In order to reduce the risk of a pneumothorax, the patient should _____ during withdrawal of the catheter.

> **Advice**
>
> **8** Look in the text about thoracentesis.
>
> **9** You are looking for a number.
>
> **10** What kind of word is missing – noun, adjective, or verb?

11 Choosing an insertion point above the _____ during thoracentesis reduces the chance of injury to the abdomen.

12 A patient may still feel tired _____ months after having pneumonia.

13 Patients who cannot _____ independently may be required to remain in hospital.

14 Patients whose blood oxygen levels are lower than _____ may be at greater risk of dying.

Advice

11 You need two words here.

12 You are looking for a number.

13 What kind of word follows 'cannot'?

14 Look in a text that is about examining the patient.

Questions 15–20

Answer each of the sentences, **15–20**, with a word or short phrase from one of the texts. Each answer may include words, numbers or both.

15 How many mls of fluid should be removed from the lung for investigation of the patient's condition?

_____

16 When performing a thoracentesis, which part of the rib should be avoided whilst inserting the needle?

_____

17 Which treatment may be necessary for patients with ARDS?

_____

18 What should be used to protect the insertion site following a thoracentesis?

_____

19 What is the risk level of a patient with a CURB65 score of 2?

_____

20 How is medication for bacteremia usually administered?

_____

Advice

15 Look in the text that gives procedures.

16 In the correct text, it tells you what the needle mustn't touch.

17 The key words here are 'ARDS' and 'treatment'.

18 This is likely to come at the end of a text.

19 Think about what CURB65 is used to determine.

20 Which text mentions bacteremia and its treatment?

Task information

- Part B tests your ability to identify the main idea, gist, purpose and to locate a specific detail within a text.

- There are six unrelated texts of 100–140 words with a three-option multiple choice question on each text.

- The question stems are either direct questions answered by one of the answer options or sentences that are completed by one of the answer options.

- The texts cover a variety of healthcare workplace text types, such as memos and emails to staff, guidelines for treatments or dealing with patients, manuals, and policy documents.

- No specialist knowledge is required to understand the texts as they are designed to be accessible to all medical professionals.

- You have 45 minutes to complete both Part B (6 questions) and Part C (16 questions).

Question focus

1   There are four main types of reading skills tested in the questions in Part B. Match the reading skills (1–4) being tested to the correct explanation (a–d) of what the reader is looking for in a text.

1 gist	**a)**	one specific piece of information given in the text
2 main idea	**b)**	the overall topic or message of the text
3 detail	**c)**	the reason the text was written (its intention)
4 purpose	**d)**	the most important point the writer is making

Main idea and detail questions

The main idea is the key message in the text and is given more emphasis, whereas a detail is one aspect of the text, often, but not necessarily related to the main idea.

1   Look at the sample Part B text (memo) below and two possible Part B question stems on the next page (without answer options) that you could be asked about it. Decide which question is asking for the main idea (M) of the text and which a specific detail (D) in the text.

To:	All staff
Subject:	Patient involvement in treatment decisions

This is a reminder that staff should facilitate the involvement of patients in treatment decisions wherever possible. This supports adherence to treatment without necessarily increasing the overall length of a consultation. Some patients may find the consultation process intimidating, so the style, speed and tone of speech should be adapted to the needs of individual patients. Any factors which could affect the patient's interpretation of explanations, such as learning disabilities or language barriers, must be considered. Avoid making assumptions about the patient's understanding and be aware of any unspoken gestures, expressions or body language which indicate that the patient wishes to make a point or does not understand what has been said. Remember that fully informed patients who have the capacity to make such decisions have the right to decide whether or not to take medication.

1 According to the memo about patient involvement in treatment decisions, it is very important for staff to ....

2 According to the memo about patient involvement in treatment decisions, one way that patients may indicate a lack of understanding is ....

2 Now look at question 1 again. Read the text. Think about the main message the writer is trying to communicate about patient involvement in treatment decisions. Write down in your own words what you think the writer's main point is.

Tip! The main idea may be stated directly or be a summary of what the writer is trying to communicate. In this text, you're looking for a summary of the message to staff.

3 Now look at the question with answer options. Which option best matches your ideas in Exercise 2 and summarises the overall message?

According to the memo about patient involvement in treatment decisions, it is very important for staff to

A make a range of adjustments to how they communicate.

B accept that poor outcomes are sometimes inevitable.

C establish whether extra support would be helpful.

4 Now look at question 2. This question stem is asking you to locate a detail in the text, specifically how patients may indicate a lack of understanding. Read the memo again. Locate and underline the section in which it mentions patient's understanding.

According to the memo about patient involvement in treatment decisions, one way that patients may indicate a lack of understanding is by …

5 Read the underlined section closely. Which way that patients may indicate their lack of understanding is mentioned? Then look at the answer options. Decide which option matches this.

A asking for advice to be repeated

B using non-verbal communication

C disregarding important information

Tip! Think about the meaning of each option rather than focusing on individual words.

Tip! All of the answer options in Part B questions are logically possible, so do not guess based on your own real life experience. Find the answer in the text.

Action plan for multiple choice questions

1 For each short text and question, quickly read the question to understand the medical context (a memo to all staff, instructions for equipment, etc.).

2 Look for and underline the locating idea(s) in the question. For example, are you reading for the main idea or specific information? It's sometimes useful to paraphrase the question in your own words as the ideas in the text will not use the same words as the options.

3 Then read the text and look for the corresponding section(s) in the text that relate to the question.

4 Underline in the text the part that answers the question and then choose the option that matches it.

5 For questions that ask you for the main idea or purpose, think about the overall message.

6 Check that the meaning in the text is a full and accurate match to the question + answer option.

Part B

In this part of the test, there are six short extracts relating to the work of health professionals. For **questions 1–6**, choose the answer (**A**, **B** or **C**) which you think fits best according to the text.

Fill the circle in completely. Example:

---

1   When first using Cough Assist, the guidelines recommend

(A)   checking that the patient is confident with the necessary technique.

(B)   giving the patient a chance to get used to the sensation it causes.

(C)   ensuring that the face covering fits the patient correctly.

> **Advice**
>
> *1 Look for a short phrase that means something is recommended.*

Extract: Cough Assist – Instructions

Cough Assist is a device that blows air into the lungs then rapidly withdraws it to clear mucus. It may need calibrating for each individual patient, in order to ensure the maximum positive (inhalation) and negative (exhalation) pressures. It is advisable to start with lower pressures, to enable the patient to become accustomed to the feel of the device. During subsequent treatments, pressures can be increased as necessary to achieve adequate secretion clearance. Note that at these lower pressures the Cough Assist may have limited effectiveness in clearing secretions.

Fix the circuit to the output, including a bacterial/viral filter, smoothbore tubing and an appropriate interface (mask, mouthpiece or trachy mount). Check starting pressures or changes in pressure requirements several times (while viewing the gauge) by blocking the circuit and having the patient rotate from inhale to exhale.

2   What does the memo say about immunoglobulin treatment?

  (A)   A lack of availability could lead to patients' therapy being revised.

  (B)   Permission may be given after administration in urgent situations.

  (C)   Patients should be advised that contracting a serious illness is unlikely.

Advice

2 The answer options all contain two ideas. In which one are both ideas covered in the text?

3 All of the ideas in the options are mentioned but two contain a word or phrase which makes them incorrect.

Memo: Patient consent and review — immunoglobulins

All treatment with immunoglobulins requires approval from the assessment panel. In the case of a clinical emergency that requires immunoglobulin for a Class II indication to be given out of hours, approval is required from the relevant on-call service.

Patients should be informed that prior consent to treatment is required. Immunoglobulins are a blood product and therefore carry an inherent low risk of blood borne infection transmission, although hepatitis A and parvovirus B19 are generally not found in clinical experience.

In the event of a supply shortage, treatment plans for long-term patients should be modified. This may include delaying treatment, switching to an alternative product, or providing an alternative treatment. Any patient whose treatment is cancelled or delayed by a duration of two weeks or more must be recorded in the incident reporting system.

---

3   What does the guideline say is the preferred approach to sterilising instruments?

  (A)   using disposable items

  (B)   purchasing an appropriate machine

  (C)   having it done by a dedicated facility

Guideline: sterilisation systems

Where possible, sterilisation should be carried out centrally using an approved local service which is bound by safeguards and supplies re-sterilised instruments. These sterile services are managed and operated by trained staff in a purpose-built environment and offer a system which is quality-controlled, cost effective and trackable.

Where such services are not available, a pre-sterilised, single-use object may be used. Advantages include convenience and suitability for use in areas where decontamination may be difficult to achieve. Alternatively, a bench top vacuum steam steriliser may be used. However, this must be installed, tested and managed appropriately according to safety regulations. It should also be noted that storage, technique and method may hinder the effectiveness of decontamination at any stage of the process.

See next page ➤

4   The main purpose of the memo about Naloxone is to

  (A) describe a variety of administration methods.

  (B) stress the importance of using it with caution.

  (C) explain why it should only be used for a brief period of time.

Advice

4 The main point or purpose of a text is often supported by examples, explanations and elaborations which may be mentioned in the answer options. Which of the answer options are main points and which ones are supporting?

5 All three options are mentioned but only one is required. Look at the three verbs at the beginning of each option to help you decide.

Memo: Naloxone use

Naloxone is an antidote to opioid drugs. It will almost immediately reverse opioid induced respiratory depression, but can counteract the analgesic effect. Staff are reminded that this rapid reversal can provoke significant adverse reactions, including intense pain, arrhythmias and even death. Use in anything other than a life-threatening emergency (respiratory arrest or profound unconsciousness) should therefore be with extreme care, starting with a low dose and gradually building up to the target dose.

The duration of Naloxone action is shorter than most opioid drugs, so careful patient observation, repeated doses or an infusion may be required to maintain clinical effect. Conversely, repeated doses without clinical effect should prompt the search for an alternative diagnosis.

5   According to the guidelines, staff are required to

  (A) submit a training certificate for the relevant technique.

  (B) verify that they have followed the correct procedure.

  (C) report any unusual findings to the relevant person.

Specimen handling guidelines:

Collection, handling and labelling of specimens has implications for microbiological diagnosis and the subsequent prescribing of antimicrobial drugs. Any staff involved with handling specimens must therefore be fully trained and competent.

In order to avoid contamination with other bacteria, protective clothing is necessary and specimens must be collected in an aseptic manner in an appropriate sterile and sealed container. A specimen laboratory form must be completed and any current or recent antibiotic prescriptions included. Care must be taken to avoid contaminating the outside of the container or forms. Results must be entered into the patients records as soon as they are available and any which are outside of normal limits should be highlighted to the patient's clinician for review and possible action. Any with infection prevention and control implications should be acted upon immediately.

6   These guidelines on switching anti-epileptic medication do not apply if

Advice

6 Again all options are mentioned but the question is asking for an exception to the guidelines.

(A)   a suitable alternative drug is stated on the prescription.

(B)   the prescription is for a condition which is not epilepsy.

(C)   no previous negative side effects have been noted.

Anti-epileptic drugs – prescribing guidelines

Following a review of spontaneous adverse reactions in patients who were switched from a branded epilepsy drug on which they were stable, to a generic one, the following guidance has been issued to help minimise risk:

*   If it is felt desirable for a patient to be maintained on a specific manufacturer's product, this should be prescribed either by specifying the brand name, or by using the generic drug name and name of the manufacturer.

*   This advice relates to antiepileptic drug use for treatment of epilepsy; it is irrelevant if their use is for other indications (e.g., mood stabilisation, neuropathic pain).

*   Please report on a Yellow Card any suspected adverse reactions to antiepileptic drugs.

*   Where possible, dispensing pharmacists should ensure the continuity of supply of a particular product when the prescription specifies it.

Task information

- You read two unrelated texts of approximately 800 words each and answer eight four-option multiple choice questions for each text.

- The texts are on medical topics but don't require specialist knowledge, and are typically articles, extracts from journals and research reviews.

- The questions are in the same order as they appear in the text and there is typically one question per paragraph, plus a reference and lexis question.

- There is typically one question per paragraph, plus a reference and a lexis question.

- Remember that you have 45 minutes to complete both Part B and Part C.

Question focus

1 The following question stems (without answer options) come from a Part C text on the origins of tuberculosis (TB). Match them to the information the question is asking you for (a–f).

1 In the first paragraph, the writer's aim is to...

2 In the second paragraph, what does the writer suggest about ideas on the origin of TB?

3 The word **'this'** in the third paragraph refers to

4 What view does the writer express when discussing Kappelman's research in the third paragraph?

5 According to the fourth paragraph, how does the writer feel about the use of genetic evidence in the study of ancient diseases?

6 The phrase **'with that information in mind'** in the fifth paragraph suggests that Oussama Baker

7 The writer refers to a skeleton found at a site called Tell Aswad in order to...

a) why the writer has referred to a particular example in the text

b) cohesion question – what a reference word refers to

c) lexical question – what a word or phrase means in context

d) the main idea of the paragraph

e) an attitude or opinion mentioned in the text

f) the writer's overall purpose in a paragraph

Opinion questions

1 Look at the second paragraph of a sample Part C text on tuberculosis (TB). Read the paragraph and answer the questions below.

Biologists long <u>thought they knew</u> where TB came from. The human pathogen is part of a group of closely related bacteria that sicken a range of animals from badgers to seals. One of these, *Mycobacterium bovis*, found commonly in cattle, can also infect humans. That is why it <u>had been assumed</u> that TB jumped to people from cattle when our ancestors domesticated them, some time after farming took off around 10,000 years ago. Evidence from ancient human remains <u>seemed to support</u> this idea. The oldest known cases of TB in Europe date from around 7000 years ago. In ancient Egypt, they date to 6500 years ago. And in China, skeletal remains point to TB being present around 6000 years ago.

1 What ideas about TB are being discussed in paragraph 2?

2 Look at the underlined sections in the text. What do they tell you about the writer's opinion of these ideas?

2 Now look at the Part C sample question and answer options. Thinking about your answers to the previous exercise, choose the correct option.

In the second paragraph, what does the writer suggest about ideas on the origins of TB in humans?

A They appear convincing but may not be true.

B They are based on facts which contradict one another.

C They prove that cross-infection frequently occurs between species.

D They show how the development of disease may be linked to location.

Tip! Opinion questions often ask you what the writer 'suggests' about the topic or part of the topic being discussed so you may need to infer opinion as it may not be stated directly.

3 Now look at the third paragraph of the text. Look at the sample opinion question. The correct answer is option B. Can you explain why?

> But in 2008, research was published that totally undermined **this**. John Kappelman at the University of Texas and his colleagues claimed to have found evidence of TB in an ancient hominin, *Homo erectus*. Diagnosing TB in ancient skeletons and fossils relies upon identifying physical abnormalities such as spinal deformity, rigidity of joints and pitting inside the skull. Kappelman and his team said they had found the last of these signs on a partial *H. erectus* skull unearthed at Kocabaş in Turkey, dating to around 500,000 years ago. Some experts find the evidence compelling. But there is much debate about the reliability of the techniques used to diagnose TB in old bones and, given the extraordinary nature of Kappelman's findings, they were unsurprisingly mostly met with scepticism.

What view does the writer express when discussing Kappelman's research in the third paragraph?

A The main strength of his study was the methodology used.

B There are good reasons why many people failed to accept his claim.

C Members of his team raised valid concerns about the procedures involved.

D The importance of his findings should have been more widely acknowledged.

Reference questions

1 The first line of paragraph 3 in the previous section contains a reference word in bold and underlined. Read the second paragraph below and then read the third paragraph again and answer the questions.

Tip! Typically, a reference word will refer back to an idea mentioned earlier in the same paragraph or text.

> Biologists long thought they knew where TB came from. The human pathogen is part of a group of closely related bacteria that sicken a range of animals from badgers to seals. One of these, *Mycobacterium bovis*, found commonly in cattle, can also infect humans. That is why it had been assumed that TB jumped to people from cattle when our ancestors domesticated them, some time after farming took off around 10,000 years ago. Evidence from ancient human remains seemed to support this idea. The oldest known cases of TB in Europe date from around 7000 years ago. In ancient Egypt, they date to 6500 years ago. And in China, skeletal remains point to TB being present around 6000 years ago.

1 Do you think 'this' refers to something in second or third paragraph?

2 Does it refer to a single idea in the paragraph you chose or the main idea?

2 Now look at the sample reference question below. Based on your answer to Exercise 1, choose the correct option.

The word **'this'** in the third paragraph refers to

A the type of bacterium which causes TB in humans.

B a physical feature indicating TB found by Kappelman.

C the date at which TB was first believed to be present in China.

D the theory that humans originally contracted TB from animals.

Attitude questions

1 Look at this sample 'attitude' question and answer options which relates to the fourth paragraph of the TB text. Underline the attitude adjective in each option and think about what the writer might say to convey this idea.

According to the fourth paragraph, how does the writer feel about the use of genetic evidence in the study of ancient diseases?

A She is concerned that it may not always be reliable.

B She is impressed by the use that Kappelman has made of it.

C She is cautious about the claims that Brosch made based on it.

D She is hopeful that it can provide additional support for earlier findings.

2 Now look at the fourth paragraph. The key ideas that indicate the attitude are underlined. Think about the adjectives from Exercise 1. Which one best matches the writer's attitude in the underlined text?

> However, the study of ancient diseases <u>needn't rely solely on this sort of evidence</u>. In recent years, a<u>dvances in genetics mean palaeopathologists can also use ancient and modern DNA to reconstruct the evolution of pathogens</u>. And <u>there is some genetic evidence suggesting that Kappelman may have been onto something</u>. A study led by Roland Brosch at the Pasteur Institute in Paris concluded that M. tuberculosis is older in origin than M. bovis, suggesting it <u>did indeed</u> evolve in humans before cattle domestication.

Tip! Attitude questions focus on determining the emotional response of the writer to something in the text.

Action plan

1 Carefully read and understand what each question is asking you for (the main idea, the purpose of what is said, why an example is used, what a reference word refers to, etc.).

2 Try to identify how the four answer options are different from each other, underlining key words such as verbs.

3 Use the clues in the question to find the relevant section in the text where the answer is found.

4 Remember the words used in the text are unlikely to be the same ones that appear in the options so read the section carefully for meaning.

5 Select your answer.

6 Check that the meaning in the text exactly and fully matches the question + answer.

Part C

In this part of the test, there are two texts about different aspects of healthcare. For **questions 7–22**, choose the answer (**A**, **B**, **C** or **D**) which you think fits best according to the text.

Fill the circle in completely. Example:

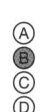

Text 1: Assisted Dying (Euthanasia)

Nowadays, many countries around the world provide exemplary standards of palliative care. However, recent research debunks the oft-cited argument that improved access to palliative care negates the need for assisted dying. There remains a significant minority of patients with fatal illnesses, whose suffering cannot be controlled, who are often denied the option of shortening their life in a dignified, swift, and painless way. I would argue that **this** should compel us to take an honest and candid look at assisted dying, carefully consider its limits, and investigate whether it can or should be a viable part of the system. Those in favour claim that it could offer a safeguard against an agonising or undignified death in cases where palliative care fails to.

Although assisted dying remains illegal in most countries, a growing number are permitting the use of what's known as the 'doctrine of double effect', whereby medication, including sedatives, can be administered to relieve a patient's symptoms in the knowledge that it could also hasten their death, providing that this is not the doctor's primary motivation. In addition, less controversial end-of-life practices, such as voluntary nil-by-mouth and withdrawal of treatment can be used. However, these practices are often a **double-edged sword**. Whilst in some cases they do provide terminally ill patients with comfortable deaths, in others the process becomes prolonged due to legal and ethical complexities. What is evident is that they carry fewer checks, balances and safeguards, yet cannot guarantee the subsequent relief of a swift death. Furthermore, research shows that more than three quarters of medical professionals consider giving the option of an assisted death more ethical than withholding treatment.

The British campaign group Dignity in Dying does not support assisted dying, but is calling for improvements to existing palliative care alongside a change in the law which would allow a terminally ill, mentally competent adult to end their own life. What seems clear is that in the absence of such a law, many dying people are taking matters into their own hands, travelling abroad for a legal assisted death or by ending their own life at home. Doctors are also stepping in to fill the void — more than six in ten healthcare professionals believe they have intentionally hastened death as a compassionate response to a patient's request to end their suffering. Many argue that it would be far safer for all involved to have a transparent law which allows assisted dying in limited circumstances with clear, upfront safeguards and monitoring.

Euthanasia is now permitted in four US states and has been legal in the Netherlands for approximately two decades. Despite concerns to the contrary, it appears that end-of-life care in these jurisdictions has improved across the board. Furthermore, there is no evidence that the practice encourages financially motivated assisted deaths. However, Theo Boer, an ethicist formerly on a Netherlands euthanasia review committee, points out that gauging patients' suffering is a subjective process, with an assisted dying law being applied in a variety of ways, depending on how the doctor in question reads it. Although Boer still favours legalisation to some extent, due to its huge democratic support, he worries that the aim of euthanasia will go from preventing a terrible death to preventing a terrible life.

In 2017, a Dutch survey found that 82% of doctors would consider a euthanasia request for a patient with a physical illness. This figure falls to approximately half that for those with psychiatric conditions or dementia, which nonetheless represents a significant proportion. The main concern surrounds such patients' lack of ability to reaffirm an advance directive. A real world example of this is the case of a Dutch doctor prosecuted for sedating and euthanising an elderly patient whilst family members restrained her. Although the patient's living will had requested it, her intellectual capacity had degraded by the time of her death and prosecutors questioned whether enough had been done to verify her consent. Clinical psychiatrist Mark Komrad cites the Netherlands as an example of how euthanasia policy can easily expand beyond its original boundaries. Nonetheless, the Dutch government continues to consider a 2016 proposal to create a complementary euthanasia law for 'people who regard their life as completed', but who are not necessarily terminally ill, a move some fear could stigmatize the elderly and undermine current euthanasia practice.

Despite fears that assisted dying could become commonplace and result in coercion and abuse, findings persistently show that this is unlikely. Those who choose it tend to be highly educated people who have thought through all the options and are very clear in their wishes. Furthermore, whist having the option of assisted dying may quell anxiety for some, it is not necessarily the most popular option. Anecdotal evidence indicates that although most patients are relieved there is an 'emergency exit', they still choose palliative care when presented with the full range of end-of-life choices.

Text 1: Questions 7–14

7 The writer uses the word '**this**' in the first paragraph to refer to

  Ⓐ sensitivity about changes to provision of end-of-life care.

  Ⓑ uncertainty about how to care for terminally ill patients .

  Ⓒ concern that end-of-life care is gradually deteriorating.

  Ⓓ distress experienced by some terminally ill patients.

8 What do we learn about the writer's attitude towards assisted dying from the first paragraph?

  Ⓐ He feels it is a topic that should be examined from all angles.

  Ⓑ He's frustrated by the amount of opposition there is to the idea.

  Ⓒ He'd like to start a debate on how to properly define the term.

  Ⓓ He is keen to see members of the public included in consultations.

9 In the second paragraph, what does the writer say about the 'doctrine of double effect'?

  Ⓐ Opposition to it is often dismissed.

  Ⓑ Its use is increasing across the world.

  Ⓒ Most people are unaware of its existence.

  Ⓓ It is more popular with some doctors than others.

10 The writer uses the phrase '**double-edged sword**' in the second paragraph to support his point that some end-of-life practices can

  Ⓐ be used to justify unethical decisions.

  Ⓑ complicate the assessment of individual cases.

  Ⓒ increase the workload of all staff involved.

  Ⓓ have both favourable and unfavourable consequences.

Tip! For reference word or vocabulary-focusing questions, the words are usually in bold and easy to find. Read the sentences immediately before and after.

Advice

7 *For this type of question, the reference word usually refers to an idea mentioned before it appears in the text.. Which answer option best summarises what he says?*

8 *The text mentions an honest and candid look. Choose the option which best summarises what he says after this.*

9 *The answer can be found in the first sentence of the paragraph.*

10 *The explanation comes after the phrase* **double-edged sword**.

Tip! All four options in the questions are designed to sound plausible.

Tip! Never rush or jump to conclusions. Find the answer in the text, not based on your opinions or experience.

See next page ▶

11 In the third paragraph the writer points out that terminally-ill patients

   Ⓐ are having to find their own solutions.

   Ⓑ are changing their perspective on death.

   Ⓒ have lost hope that a solution will be found.

   Ⓓ fear being put at risk by unqualified practitioners.

12 According to Theo Boer, one of the risks of legalising assisted dying is that

   Ⓐ not all doctors will interpret such a law in the same way.

   Ⓑ the autonomy of doctors could be put at risk.

   Ⓒ it could be difficult to reverse if public opinion changes.

   Ⓓ It may lead to reduced levels of public trust in the medical profession.

13 In the fifth paragraph, the writer uses the example of the court case in the Netherlands to show how

   Ⓐ cognitive decline can complicate the interpretation of a person's wishes.

   Ⓑ quickly families reverse decisions on behalf of terminally ill patients.

   Ⓒ determined the Dutch government was to legalise assisted dying.

   Ⓓ little public support there is for assisted dying for mentally ill patients.

14 What opinion about assisted dying does the writer express in the final paragraph?

   Ⓐ Certain portions of society may never see it as an acceptable choice.

   Ⓑ Concerns which surround it are not fully supported by evidence.

   Ⓒ Demand for it will increase as soon as initial problems are resolved.

   Ⓓ A great deal of work is needed to persuade people of the need for it.

Advice

11 Remember that the question is asking about patients are doing or feel.

12 This question focuses on what Theo Boer says, not the writer's opinion.

13 Scan the paragraph for the section which discusses the court case. How does the writer introduce the case?

14 Check that all the ideas in the answer options are represented in the text.

See next page ▶

Text 2: Should obesity be classed as a disease?

Driven by powerful cultural and economic factors, obesity is widely recognised as one of the most important health issues facing the world today. Prevalence has tripled over the past forty years, raising it to epidemic proportions, with more than 13 percent of the world's adult population classified as obese. Although largely avoidable, obesity is a major risk factor for an alarming number of potentially fatal non-communicable conditions, such as cardiovascular disease (the leading global cause of death in 2019), diabetes, musculoskeletal disorders and some cancers. Prevalence in the UK is expected to hit 35 percent by 2030. This is a daunting figure, as obesity not only places a heavy strain on the healthcare system, but also damages educational outcomes, labour force productivity and the economy.

The World Health Organisation (WHO) defines obesity as 'abnormal or excessive fat accumulation that may impair health' and have classed it as a disease since 1936. Calls for the UK to follow suit are increasing. Proponents claim that reclassification would inevitably lead to increased funds being allocated to fighting it, allowing for more research into its behavioural, environmental and genetic causes. This in turn would lead to the development of more effective healthcare policies, ranging all the way from prevention, to medical and surgical treatments. **This is already the case** for other 'recognised' diseases which are related to lifestyle choices, such as COPD or lung cancer in a person who smokes. Moreover, it would encourage people to discuss their condition and seek treatment. Stigmatisation and humiliation frequently leave patients fearful of doing so, causing some to turn to futile fad diets or unsafe non-prescription medication.

The popular view is that obesity is self-inflicted and a consequence of being 'weak-willed', but findings suggest that this assumption may be incorrect. Studies in twins show that 40–70% of variability in weight is inherited and that body weight and fat distribution are strongly influenced by genetic make-up. After all, our genes contain the programming to send the body instructions for responding to important changes, for example, by increasing appetite and food intake, all of which implies that there is a significant genetic component to obesity.

One further possible advantage of classifying obesity as a disease is that it could eventually lead to governments tackling **the elephant in the room**, namely that socio-economic factors are key drivers. Income, housing, education, access to space and exposure to the advertising and sale of unhealthy foods all impact on how active we are and whether we can eat healthily and until now, this fact has been wilfully ignored. Unfortunately for one in five people eating healthily is a luxury they cannot afford. Access to healthy food should be an entitlement, rather than a privilege, yet adults in the most deprived areas of the UK are almost twice as likely to be obese as those in the least deprived areas. This gap is even more pronounced in children and appears to be widening.

Dr Agnes Ayton believes that the 'cafeteria diet' may be at least partly to blame for the current obesogenic environment and research supports this view. The metabolic effects of processed foods we eat today have been studied in animals. Replacing their standard diet with such a diet leads to hyperphagia (overeating), resulting in dramatic weight gain. Such experimental data is analogous to the human experience. A recent groundbreaking randomised controlled trial found that the hunger hormone ghrelin rises when an ultra-processed diet is consumed, leading to bingeing and overeating through altering multiple endocrine pathways.

Recognising obesity as a disease could help facilitate a much-needed shift from our current obesogenic tendencies, but not everyone agrees. Dr Richard Pile warns that it could result in even worse outcomes for both individuals and society and cautions against encouraging fatalism and promoting the fallacy that our BMI is predetermined. He claims that the recommendation risks reducing autonomy and eliminating the intrinsic motivation that is an important enabler of change. He is also wary of the implication that current strategies are doomed to failure and that labelling obesity as a disease represents the missing piece in the jigsaw puzzle. The Oxford Dictionary defines a disease as 'a disorder of structure or function', which, Pile argues, is so vague that we can classify almost anything as one. The question is not whether we can, but whether we should, and to what end.

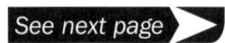
See next page

Text 1: Questions 15–22

15 What is the writer doing in the first paragraph?

(A) criticising current attitudes towards obese people

(B) explaining why obesity is linked to so many chronic diseases

(C) emphasising the negative impact obesity has on society as a whole

(D) pointing out the difficulties involved in predicting future levels of obesity

16 In the second paragraph the writer argues that classifying obesity as a disease would

(A) cause some people's anxiety about their weight to worsen.

(B) deter patients from exploring potentially harmful remedies.

(C) lead to excessive numbers of patients trying to access services.

(D) have little effect on feelings of shame associated with the condition.

17 What is the writer referring to with the phrase '**this is already the case**' in the second paragraph?

(A) the positive impact of better resourcing

(B) an increased focus on preventative measures

(C) the combined efforts of committed individuals

(D) an improved understanding of how a problem arose

18 What is the writer's attitude towards the twin studies mentioned in the third paragraph?

(A) It is hard to understand why it has taken so long for them to be carried out.

(B) It's disappointing that people aren't more curious about them.

(C) Further research is needed to confirm the findings.

(D) The conclusions they came to are hardly surprising.

Advice

15 Think about the overall message of the paragraph.

16 Again, focus on the verbs that begin each option. Which best describes the overall effect reclassification would have?

17 Be careful! One of the incorrect options is mentioned in the text, but it is only one aspect of what 'this' refers.

18 Think about the phrase 'After all' and why it is used.

19 What is the writer highlighting when he refers to socio-economic factors as 'the elephant in the room', in the fourth paragraph?

(A) the opposition faced by those who attempt to bring the topic into the open

(B) the discomfort people feel when they are asked to discuss such issues

(C) the sensitivity needed when trying to understand their impact

(D) the reluctance of those in power to address the role they play

20 In the fourth paragraph, the writer suggests that healthy food choices are

(A) beyond the reach of certain sections of the population.

(B) rarely prioritised by the majority of consumers.

(C) heavily influenced by parental attitudes.

(D) unappealing to many modern families.

21 What does the research into 'cafeteria diet' say leads to overeating?

(A) Lack of independent research into impacts of convenience foods.

(B) Food choices being controlled by underlying eating disorders.

(C) People consuming foods which stimulate the appetite.

(D) Manufacturers putting addictive ingredients in food.

22 What view does Dr Richard Pile express about obesity in the sixth paragraph?

(A) Encouraging changes in lifestyle may eventually resolve the issue.

(B) Removing personal responsibility could compound the problem.

(C) Existing approaches to the problem are likely to be ineffective.

(D) Exploring new solutions will probably be a waste of resources.

Task information

- The Writing test is 45 minutes long.
- You have to write a formal letter of about 180–200 words to another medical professional about a patient.
- The letter is specific and relevant to your medical profession and is either a letter of referral, discharge or transfer.
- The first five minutes of the test is for you to read the task and some corresponding case notes, and the remaining 40 minutes is for you to write your letter. You are not allowed to make any notes during the first five minutes of the test.
- To write your letter, you will need to select and organise the information from the case notes that is relevant to the type of letter you are being asked to write.
- You are provided with a separate Answer Booklet to write your letter into.

How the letter is assessed

Your letter is assessed against six criteria (see page 212 for more details). Study them to understand what your mark depends on.

1 Below are five questions you should cover in order to score highly in the writing task. Match them to the following three assessment criteria for the letter: **Purpose (P)**, **Content (C)** and **Organisation and Layout (O)**. Use the information on page 212 if necessary.

   1 Are my paragraphs logically sequenced and coherent for the reader? ....

   2 Does my letter contain everything the reader needs to know for the patient's continued care? ....

   3 Does my letter make it clear to the reader why it was written and what they are expected to do next? ....

   4 Is the key information presented in a way that makes it easy for the reader to locate and understand? ....

   5 Is all the information included in the letter accurate? ....

Identifying the target reader and purpose of the letter

Use the planning time to identify the purpose and target reader and think about what the reader needs to know to continue care for the patient. Consider the letter type (discharge, referral or transfer), the reader's job function and role in the patient's recovery, and whether they already know the patient.

> **Tip!** A referral will typically require further investigation, diagnosis, tests or treatment of your patient. Discharge or transfer letters typically hand over care of the patient to the reader, so the focus is on providing information related to continued care.

1 Look at these common target readers in OET Writing and complete the sentences about their job function with verbs from the box in the correct form.

| improve | provide | prevent | perform | recommend | identify | assess | organise |

Reader	Role in continued care
Dietitian	A dietitian **(1)** .... changes in food and nutrition to help **(2)** .... the patient's condition and **(3)** .... further disease.
A surgeon	A surgeon **(4)** .... a preoperative diagnosis of the patient, and then **(5)** .... the operation, and ensures that the patient has adequate postoperative care.
Social worker	A social worker **(6)** .... a person's social and interpersonal needs, strengths and preferences and helps **(7)** .... support and services they need to solve their problems.
Community nurse	A community nurse works in a specific setting, like a health centre, care home or even visiting people in their own homes, to **(8)** .... their healthcare needs and provide treatment.

2 Look at these two Writing tasks and for each circle the target reader and underline the purpose of the letter you are being asked to write.

Tip! It's a good idea to start your letter by stating the purpose for the target reader in the opening paragraph.

1 Using the information in the case notes, write a referral letter to the dietitian, Ms Amanda Hart, outlining Ms Rogers' relevant history and current problem. Her address is Newtown Clinic, 111 High Street, Newtown.

2 Using the information in the case notes, write a letter of transfer to the orthopaedic clinic at Newtown Hospital requesting definitive diagnosis and surgical treatment. Address your letter to the surgeon, Dr Jim Harley, Orthopaedic Clinic, 36 Hadley Close, Newtown Hospital.

Organising your letter and selecting appropriate content

You need to pick out the key information from the case notes and then organise it into logical paragraphs. Not everything in the case notes is required.

1 Now look at this extract from the patient's case notes that accompany the writing task. The information has been numbered 1–16. Look at the two writing tasks in the previous exercise in the previous section, and decide for each piece of information whether it is relevant to the Dietician task (D), Surgeon (S), both tasks (B) or neither (N). Give reasons.

Notes:

Patient name:	Ms Zoe Rogers
DOB:	24 January, 1980 (41 y.o.)
Social background:	Investment banker **(1)** .... No exercise **(2)** .... Smokes: 2 cigs/day **(3)** .... Diet: Vegetarian; convenience meals, eats out 4x/wk; 6–7 cups coffee/day **(4)** ....
Medical history:	2019: Diag. w diabetes mellitus type 2 **(5)** .... 500mg metformin 2x/day **(6)** ....

Emergency Department Admission: 24 January, 2021

Presenting problem:	R distal forearm swelling, visible deformity **(7)** .... L knee deep cut – tripped over rock **(8)** ....
Diagnosis:	?Low trauma R wrist Colles fracture - ?osteopenia cause of fracture **(9)** ....
Tests:	AP, Oblique, Lateral X-rays: Displaced, dorsally angulated distal radius fracture **(10)** .... FBC, TSH: Normal **(11)** .... BMD: Z score <−2 (low bone density = osteopenia) **(12)** .... Total Serum 25-hydroxyvitamin D: 12 ng/mL (moderate deficiency – ? osteopenia secondary factor) **(13)** ....
Plan:	Supplement w D2: 50,000 IUs/wk **(14)** .... Refer dietitian: Recommend Vitamin D-rich food; 'easy to cook' meals **(15)** .... Transfer to orthopaedic clinic to treat R fracture = ?Open reduction internal fixation (ORIF surgery) **(16)** ....

2 Look at the student's notes about what topics (a–d) to include in their letters for the Writing tasks in the previous section. For each task, decide on a logical order to present the topics in the respective letters and how to paragraph the information.

To surgeon		To dietitian
a) relevant tests		a) relevant social background
b) future needs		b) summary of diagnosis
c) summary of presenting complaint and provisional diagnosis		c) current problem and relevant tests
		d) future needs

3 Read two possible paragraphs about the patient's 'relevant social background' for the dietitian writing task. Which one best highlights key information for the target reader and why?

Paragraph A: Ms. Rogers is a vegetarian and prefers to eat convenience meals, and usually eats out 4 times a week. She does not consume alcohol but drinks about 6–7 cups of coffee a day. She smokes 2 cigarettes daily and does not exercise.

Paragraph B: Ms. Rogers smokes 2 cigarettes daily and does not exercise. She does not drink alcohol but drinks 6–7 cups of coffee a day. She prefers to eat convenience meals and eats out 4 times a week. She is a vegetarian.

4 Now read two possible paragraphs about the patient's future needs for the surgeon writing task and decide which one best highlights key information for the reader.

Paragraph A: Ms Rogers has been prescribed 50,000 IUs of supplemental Vitamin D weekly and she has been referred to a dietitian for recommendations of vitamin D-rich foods. It would be appreciated if you could provide immediate treatment of her low trauma right wrist fracture at the orthopaedic clinic, performing open reduction internal fixation (ORIF surgery) as required.

Paragraph B: It would be appreciated if you could provide immediate treatment of her low trauma right wrist fracture at the orthopaedic clinic, performing open reduction internal fixation (ORIF surgery) as required.

Tip! The order of the information in the case notes is not necessary the best order to present it in your letter. Try to make key information for the reader prominent at the start of paragraphs.

Action plan

Before you write

- Use the first five minutes to read the case notes and writing task but remember that you cannot make notes, underline or highlight anything.
- Identify the purpose and target reader for your letter.
- Consider which information should be included or omitted.
- Think carefully about how you will divide the information in the case notes into logical paragraphs based on the task.
- Use the above to make a paragraph plan once the reading time is up. This will help ensure that your letter is coherent and contains all the relevant information.

As you write

- Use the features formal letter format throughout including address details of the reader, the date, and ensure that your language is appropriate.

- Make sure that the purpose of your letter is clear in the first paragraph.
- Make sure the purpose of each paragraph is clear with key information prioritised and accurately expressed.
- Use linking words and phrases or sequence, addition, contrast, and cause and effect to make your paragraphs easy to follow for the reader (e.g., *In addition*; *Finally*; *Therefore*; *Nevertheless*, etc.).

After you write

- When you have finished, read through your letter for clarity, and to correct any mistakes which typically can occur under exam conditions, especially common errors that you make when writing.

TIME ALLOWED: READING TIME: 5 MINUTES
                   WRITING TIME: 40 MINUTES

Read the case notes and complete the writing task which follows.

Notes:

Assume that today's date is 10 July 2020.

You are a family doctor at Hightown Medical Clinic where a mother has brought in her young child to see you.

PATIENT DETAILS:

Name:	Molly Smith (Miss)
DOB:	23 June 2017 (3 y.o.)
Address:	1001 Hightown Way, Hightown
Medical history:	All vaccines up to date Eczema: flexor surfaces, arms & legs (occasional, treatment = topical corticosteroid cream)
Family History:	Nil significant
Social Background:	Mother = homemaker Father = plumber 2 older sisters (5 y.o. & 7 y.o.) Cared for by maternal grandmother 2x/wk (mother needs support)
Allergies:	No known allergies

Hospital Treatment Record:

Presentation at ED:

3 July 2020

Mother reported: pt pulled tablecloth, pot w hot water fell & scolded her

Diagnosis:

2nd degree partial thickness burns, 18% of TBSA (total body surface area): face, hands, arms & trunk

Treatment:
Admssion to ICU
IV fluid & pain relief
Move to burns unit (further management)

Burns Unit:

5 July 2020

Progress: pain level reported = 8/10

FBC: sepsis ruled out

Treatment: surgical debridement & grafting to ↓mortality

8 July 2020

Healing well
Pain level reported = 4/10
Pt ready for discharge

Requires pressure garments, sponge bath, no swimming
Paracetamol 5 ml oral suspension 4x/day
Note: outpatient clinic appt 13 July (dressing change)

Presentation at Hightown Medical Clinic:

9 July 2020

Pt & mother attend: mother reports pt's general lethargy & some distress
Pain reported as 5/10
Mother compliant w. discharge plan (pressure garments, sponge bath, medication)
Asked to return if symptoms persist

10 July 2020

Subjective: ↑pain (6/10), itchiness at burns site
Mother reports: worsening overnight, disorientation, unsteadiness on feet (trip hazards removed), pt fell over dog →bleeding at burns site

Objective: temp 38.5°C, burns site red & warm to touch
Topical antiseptic applied, burns site redressed
Antibiotics prescribed
?infection
?sepsis

Plan:

Urgent referral to hospital burns unit

Writing Task:

Using the information in the case notes, write a letter of referral to Dr Mayfield, Plastic Surgeon, outlining your concerns about the patient and requesting urgent investigation, definitive diagnosis and further management. Address the letter to Dr Scarlett Mayfield, Plastic Surgeon, Outpatient Burns Unit, Hightown Hospital, 123 High Street, Hightown.

Tip! Identify what information in the case notes should be included based on the target reader and purpose of the letter.

Tip! Case notes abbreviations should be familiar to you and more unfamiliar abbreviations will be explained in the brackets.

In your answer:
- **Expand the relevant notes into complete sentences**
- **Do not use note form**
- **Use letter format**

The body of the letter should be approximately 180–200 words.

Task information

- You hear audio extracts from two consultations between patients and healthcare professionals each of about five minutes in length.

- The healthcare professionals may not be from your own profession, but no specialist knowledge is needed to follow what is being said.

- For each extract, you need to complete 12 gaps in a set of patient notes that correspond to what is said. The patient notes follow the order that the information you listen for appears in the audio extract.

- You have to write a word or short phrase you hear in the audio extract to complete the gaps.

- The missing information typically comes from the patient not the medical professional.

- Before each recording, you have 30 seconds to read the patient notes and two minutes at the end to check your answers for both sets of notes.

- You hear each extract only once.

Using patient notes to understand structure and content of consultations

Before listening, familiarise yourself with the patient notes to understand the structure/direction of the consultation This helps you anticipate what you will hear and what the missing information might be.

1 Look at these examples of context sentences that introduce the patient notes. For each, underline the medical professional and then make notes on the types of conditions/injuries they might treat.

   1 You hear a dermatologist talking to a new patient called Lucy Clarke.

   2 You hear an opthalmologist talking to a patient called Nathan Bridges.

2 Look at the table below which contains a list of common sub-headings in patient notes and two medical professional roles. Complete the table with words or phrases from the box that might correspond to each sub-heading and role.

> **Tip!** Each set of patient notes is different, so you will see different subheadings in each task.

| CT scan | itchy | vision loss | Triptan p.r.n | sudden | ESR | severe headaches |
| rash | eye pain | appearance of skin | risk of infection | MRI | topical corticosteroid |

Sub-headings	Neurologist	Dermatologist
Background to condition	started 3 weeks ago, same time every day (early morning)	psoriasis diagnosed 18 months ago
Onset of symptoms / current symptoms	......................, ..., ...	......................, ..., severe sunburn
Diagnosis and treatment	....	....
Tests / Investigations	......................, ...	......................, biopsy
Patient concerns	worsening pain, ...	......................, ...

Anticipating the missing information

Each sub-heading in the patient notes contains bullet points, some of which are gapped and need to be completed. Read the notes before you listen to anticipate what you are listening for.

1 Look at the context sentence, sub-headings, and gapped bullet points below. For each, decide which of the two options in brackets makes the most sense in the gap and explain why.

You hear a dermatologist talking to a new patient called Lucy Clarke.

Onset of symptoms	• appearance of skin – red and flaky with **(1)** .... (*silvery scales / severe*)
	• intense **(2)** .... (*food / stress*)
Current medication	• **(3)** .... p.r.n. (*antihistamine / discontinued*)
Patient concerns	• patches may be **(4)** .... (*spreading / reducing*)
Patient requests	• wants to receive **(5)** .... (*specialist / phototherapy*)

Tip! The missing information in each gap is often a noun or noun phrase related to the conditions/symptoms/ treatments, though sometimes it could be an adjective or verb.

Listening for cues in the audio

As you follow the notes, listen out for words and phrases the patient uses that match the ideas in the notes as these signal that the information you need to listen for is coming.

1 The following phrases from the audio extract are cues for the missing information in the notes below. Match the audio cues (a–f) to the sub-headings and bullets in the notes (1–6).

a) '*It covers quite a big area – it's all over my...*'

b) '*Not only that, but it hurts too. I can't stop scratching it, and it's so ...*'

c) '*It looks awful... It's red... and there are flakes.. and it has these ...*'

d) '*... the joints in my lower legs and feet – they were kind of puffy and ...*'

e) '*I had no idea that they were connected. I thought I had a new, completely different problem. I noticed that ...*'

f) '*From the age of about eight to 15 I did have to deal with ...*'

Tip! The words used in the audio may be similar to those in the bullets, but not an exact match, and usually the information is expressed in a different way.

Background to psoriasis	• Childhood **(1)** .... (until age 15)
Ongoing symptoms	• appearance – red and flaky with **(2)** ....
	• painful – itchy and **(3)** ....
	• large, constant patches on **(4)** ...., face and neck
Recent symptoms	• pitted **(5)** ...., separating from beds
	• ankles, knees and toes **(6)** .... and swollen

2  Now listen to the audio extract for the patient notes in Exercise 1. Complete gaps 1–6 with a word or short phrase.

Tip! Often the medical professional speaks when the conversation is moving onto a different sub-heading in the notes so pay attention to what they say to help you follow the audio.

Action plan

Before listening

1 Read the context sentence and look at the sub-headings to see what the conversation is about and how it is organised and develops.

2 Skim the bullet points in each section to find out the subject and details of the consultation.

3 Use the context to anticipate the kind of answer required for each gap (e.g., name of condition, medicine or treatment, adjective for describing symptoms, number, etc.) and think of potential answers.

While listening

1 Follow the recording in the case notes and write your answers as you listen.

2 Use the sub-headings to help you decide which answer you are listening for next. Don't panic if you realise you have missed an answer. Keep listening and answering and return to the missing answer at the end.

3 You will hear the exact word(s) for each gap, so do not change the form of words you hear.

4 If you are unsure of an answer, note down what you think it is and return to it at the end.

After listening

1 Use the two minutes at the end of the listening test to check that your answers are legible and makes grammatical sense in the context.

2 Make sensible guesses for any answers you missed or are unsure of, based on what you remember of the conversation.

Part A

  In this part of the test, you'll hear two different extracts. In each extract, a health professional is talking to a patient.

For **questions 1–24**, complete the notes with information you hear.

Now, look at the notes for extract one.

Extract 1: Questions 1–12

You hear a cardiologist talking to a patient called Bryn Turnbull. For **questions 1–12**, complete the notes with a word or short phrase that you hear.

You now have thirty seconds to look at the notes.

Patient: Bryn Turnbull

Onset of condition (four years ago)

- started to become more aware of his heartbeat

    – describes heartbeat as **(1)** _____
      (intermittent)

    – no accompanying pain or **(2)** _____

    – unrelated to time of day or level of activity

- no treatment initially

    n.b. father died from heart disease (following
    (3) _____ surgery)

Development of symptoms (two years ago)

- single instance of tachycardia - describes heart as
  (4) _____

    – occurred whilst **(5)** _____ (relatively
      light exercise)

- referral to cardiologist – arrhythmia confirmed by holter monitor

- mild mitral valve regurgitation identified

    – (probably present since **(6)** _____)

Medication

- prescribed low-dose beta-blockers – taken as needed

    (approx. **(7)** ___ _____ in six months)

    – **(8)** _____ and coldness in extremities
      as side effects

    – noticeably **(9)** _____ after taking his
      medication

Current symptoms

- recent overseas trip resulted in diagnosis of suspected

    (10) _____

- has developed intermittent pain in shoulders

    – radiating to neck and **(11)** _____

    – pain presents as a **(12)** _____

Extract 2: Questions 13–24

You hear a primary-care physician talking to a new patient called Jason Weiss. For **questions 13–24**, complete the notes with a word or short phrase that you hear.

You now have thirty seconds to look at the notes.

Patient: Jason Weiss

Onset of condition
- bad cold developed into a chest infection (eighteen months ago)
- breathing difficulties – **(13)** _____ sensation in chest
- left with a persistent **(14)** _____
- unintended weight loss
- subsequent difficulty **(15)** _____ and acid reflux (night time)
- diagnosed with **(16)** _____ and mild GERD

Pulmonology referral
- **(17)** _____ and early stage pulmonary fibrosis ruled out
- **(18)** _____ identified in lungs – mild COPD diagnosed
- reports being a **(19)** _____ in childhood

Current symptoms
- joint pain – initially in **(20)** _____ – but now more widespread
- treated with analgesia plus **(21)** _____
- sedentary lifestyle – works as a

  (22) _____
- n.b. fractured femur in skiing accident – closed reduction (5 years ago)

Family history
- father deceased (emphysema)
- maternal grandmother had **(23)** _____
- mother recently diagnosed with

  (24) _____

Task information

- You hear six short extracts and answer one three-option multiple-choice question on each extract.
- Each extract focuses on everyday workplace communication in a different healthcare setting, for example, staff briefings, patient handovers, etc.
- Each extract has either one or two speakers.
- Each extract lasts for about 45 seconds and you hear it once.

- You don't need any specialist knowledge to answer the questions.
- Each question has a different focus, for example, you may need to listen for detail, for the speaker's main point or for what needs to happen next in terms of patient care.
- The question stems can be either direct questions with three answer options or be sentences that are completed by one of the three options.

Preparing to listen

Each Part B question has three parts: a context sentence that tells you what you're going to hear, a question stem that tells you what you're being asked to listen for, and three answer options. Use the time before you listen to think about the context and the particular focus of each question.

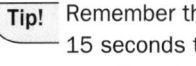 **Tip!** Remember that you have 15 seconds to read each question stem and options before you listen.

1 Look at these context sentences. What are you going to hear? Complete the first two columns of the table. The first one has been done for you.

  1 You hear a physiotherapist briefing his new assistant on post-operative care for one patient group.

  2 You hear a doctor giving feedback to a junior colleague whose work he's supervising.

  3 You hear a hospital nurse talking to a patient about arrangements for his discharge

  4 You hear a briefing for staff in a primary-care practice about a new online prescription service.

Who is speaking	Context / topic
(1) physiotherapist / new assistant	post-op care for a specific group of patients
(2)	
(3)	
(4)	

2 The question stem tells you more about what you're going to hear and help you decide exactly what you're listening for. Look at these context sentences and the question stem. What are you listening for? Choose a) or b).

  1 You hear a physiotherapist briefing his new assistant about post-operative care for one patient group. What is he emphasising about the patients?

    a) a description of the different stages of post-operative care.

    b) something related to patient care that the new assistant should be aware of.

  2 You hear a doctor giving feedback to a junior colleague whose work she's supervising. What aspect of the procedure he observed could be improved?

    a) a problem that arose and was effectively dealt with.

    b) a problem that arose that should have been avoided.

3 You hear a hospital nurse briefing her colleague about a patient. What does she warn him about?

    a) something about the patient that the colleague needs to know/be careful about/avoid

    b) the consequences of something that the colleague has done wrong.

4 You hear a hospital nurse talking to a colleague about a patient. What does she need help with?

    a) reasons why her workload is especially heavy today

    b) an aspect of patient care the nurse is unable to deal with on her own

3 The answer options all refer to things you hear about in the recording, but only one answers the question you've been asked. Look at the following two question stems with the answer options. Underline the key words in the question and options. Question 1 has been done for you as an example.

  1 You hear a physiotherapist briefing his new assistant about post-operative care for one patient group. What <u>aspect</u> of <u>patient care</u> is he <u>emphasising</u>?

    A the <u>importance</u> of using a <u>non-judgemental approach</u>

    B the <u>difficulty</u> in <u>keeping</u> these <u>patients motivated</u>

    C the <u>challenge</u> that <u>certain movements</u> may represent <u>for patients</u>

  2 You hear a doctor giving feedback to a junior colleague whose work she's supervising.

    What aspect of the procedure he observed could be improved?

    A responding to patient anxieties

    B precision in the technique itself

    C dealing with unexpected problems

4 Look again at the options for the two questions in Exercise 3. Which idea (i–vi) matches what you might hear about in the recording if each of the options was correct? The first one has been done for you.

    i) something is mentioned that hadn't been planned for, which had negative consequences *Question 2 Option C*

    ii) specific patient physical difficulties or mobility issues

    iii) how keen patients are to engage with aspects of their care.

    iv) the need to deal with a specific patient's concerns in a reassuring way

    v) the need to deal with patients' concerns in general in a reassuring way

    vi) details of how a procedure was incorrectly performed

Tip! Be careful! Sometimes the correct answer option might relate to a particular piece of information expressed in the recording and sometimes it might relate to the recording as a whole.

5  Now listen and answer the questions in Exercise 3. Then check the Answer Key for a detailed explanation.

Action plan

Before listening

1 Before listening to each extract, read and understand the introduction sentence, question and answer options.

2 Underline the key words of the question that you need to listen for.

3 Underline the key ideas in the answer options which make them different from each other.

While listening

1 Listen to the recording focusing on meaning, rather than listening for individual words in the answer options.

2 Select the answer option which best matches the meaning of what you hear even if it uses different words or expressions.

3 Record your answer clearly by filling in the correct option.

4 Make sure you have answered each question and make your best guess if unsure.

Part B

In this part of the test, you'll hear six different extracts. In each extract, you'll hear people talking in a different healthcare setting.

For **questions 25–30**, choose the answer (**A**, **B** or **C**) which fits best according to what you hear. You'll have time to read each question before you listen. Complete your answers as you listen.

Now look at question 25.

Fill the circle in completely. Example:

---

25 You hear a senior hospital nurse briefing her team about some guidelines.

The document she's talking about deals with

(A) a new policy that is being introduced.

(B) a health issue that may affect members of staff.

(C) an aspect of patient care that needs particular attention.

Advice

25 Focus on who the guidelines are for.

26 You hear a doctor talking to a medical student who's going to observe her consultation with a patient.

Why has the patient come to see the doctor?

- (A) He's been having some issues following surgery.

- (B) He's experiencing some new symptoms.

- (C) He's due for a routine health check.

27 You hear two hospital nurses conducting a patient handover.

What does the incoming nurse agree to do for the patient?

- (A) arrange for her to see a specialist

- (B) ensure that she has intravenous hydration

- (C) talk to her about possible triggers for her condition

28 You hear a community nurse visiting an elderly patient in his home.

She's going to suggest a reassessment of the patient's

- (A) mobility needs.

- (B) skin integrity.

- (C) leg injury.

Advice

26 You won't hear the words in the answer options in the recording, but you will hear the name of a type of surgery, some symptoms and another way of saying 'routing check.' Listen to what the doctor says about these things.

27 The 'incoming' nurse is mostly listening and saying 'OK', 'right' and 'sure' to show that he's understood. One of these responses refers to something he agrees to do. Listen for when the other nurse suggests asking about something again.

28 The patient makes a request that the nurse will refer him to the doctor. Listen for what it's regarding.

29 You hear part of an induction programme for new members of clinical staff at a hospital.

The session on electronic medical records is going to focus on

(A) familiarisation with the system.

(B) how to avoid errors in the system.

(C) linking medical devices to the system.

30 You hear part of a briefing meeting for staff in a local health centre.

The patient being discussed needs nursing help to learn how to

(A) change her own dressings.

(B) self-administer her medication.

(C) cope with her activities of daily living.

Advice

29 The speaker talks about all three ideas mentioned in the options – but he indicates the main focus when he says: 'So that's our aim today.'

30 Read the question carefully. The patient who's being discussed needs help with all three things at the moment, but what does she need help to 'learn to do'?

Task information

- You hear two longer extracts on different topics and you answer six questions on each.
- Each extract lasts for about five minutes and you hear it once only.
- You have 90 seconds preparation time to read the questions before you hear each extract.
- Each extract is about a different healthcare topic, but you don't need specialist medical knowledge.

- Each extract may be either an interview or a presentation.
- The question stems are either direct questions with three answer options or sentences that are completed by one of the three options.
- Each question refers to one section of the recording and the questions follow the order of the interview or presentation.

Listening for cues and key words

Use the preparation time before each extract to read the context sentence, the question stems and the answer options so that you understand how each recording is structured and what you're listening for in each question.

1 Look at the sample context sentences for Part C extracts. For each, identify how many speakers you will hear, the profession of the main speaker and the topic being discussed.

1 You hear an interview with a nurse educator called Marika Alford, who's talking about a project to help student nurses develop the skills associated with delivering bad news.

2 You hear an interview with an occupational therapist called Gabriel de la Cruz, who's talking about helping children to develop fine motor skills.

3 You hear an emergency nurse called Kofi Everard giving a presentation about giving a presentation about ways of managing the patient journey in hospital.

2 Look again at context sentence 1 from Exercise 1 with the six question stems (without answer options). Match each question stem to the sub-topics that you think will be spoken about in the recording (a–f). The first one has been done for you as an example.

You hear an interview with a nurse educator called Marika Alford, who's talking about a project to help student nurses develop the skills associated with delivering bad news.

1 What does Marika identify as the main role of nurses in the delivery of bad news to patients? c

2 Marika's team decided to set up the project on delivering bad news as a result of

3 Marika feels that student nurses receive little training in delivering bad news because

4 Why did Marika's team decide to use simulations as part of the project?

5 What aspect of the training did Marika find surprisingly successful?

6 What does Marika feel that the most worthwhile aspect of the training for students was?

a) the main benefit for those taking part in the project

b) how well (or badly) one aspect of the project went

c) the background to the project

d) the reason why the project chose a certain technique, strategy or solution

e) the cause of a problem/issue that the project was trying to address

f) what led to the development of the project

 Tip! Part C extracts often cover aspects of the main topic such these. Other common sub-topics could include the views/experiences of different people, future implications and the next steps in a project.

3  When you listen to the recording, you often hear 'cues' from the speakers which tell you that they're moving onto a new aspect of the main topic and a new question in the task. Listen to the following cues for the recording about Marika Alford's training project. Decide which question each cue refers to. Note down any words that help you decide. The first one has been done for you as an example.

Tip! As this extract is an interview, the cues all come from the interviewer. In a presentation, there is only one speaker, but you can still expect to hear the cues.

Question	Audio cue	Key words
1 What does Marika identify as the main role of nurses in the delivery of bad news to patients?		
2 Marika's team decided to set up the project on delivering bad news as a result of	1	led you to set up
3 Marika feels that student nurses receive little training in delivering bad news because		
4 Why did Marika's team decide to use simulations as part of the project		
5 What aspect of the training did Marika find surprisingly successful?		
6 Marika feels that the most worthwhile aspect of the training for students was?		

4 Use the preparation time to read through and underline key ideas in the question stem and options, so you know what you're listening for in the recording. Look at questions 1 and 2 with the answer options. For question 1, the key ideas are underlined. Underline the key ideas in question 2.

1 What does Marika <u>identify</u> as the <u>main role of nurses</u> in the delivery of bad news to patients?

   A <u>supporting</u> <u>other health</u> professionals in the task
   B doing any <u>follow-up work with patients and families</u>
   C ensuring that it's always <u>done</u> in the most <u>appropriate way</u>

2 Marika's team decided to set up the project on delivering bad news as a result of

   A being asked to cover the topic in their classes.
   B realising that they'd all had similar experiences of it.
   C discovering how badly it was dealt with on some courses.

5    Now listen to the beginning of the recording where the two questions in Exercise 4 are addressed. Choose the correct answer option for each question.

Tip! Listen for ideas that match the ideas in the options in relation to the question. We will look at this in more depth in Test 2 Training.

Action plan

Before listening	While listening
Before listening	**While listening**
1 Read and understand the introduction sentence, so you can start thinking about the topic.	1 Listen carefully to the recording for the answers to each question.
2 Look at the questions to understand the form and direction of the interview/talk.	2 Select the answer option which best matches the meaning of what is said and answers the question.
3 Underline the key idea in the questions.	3 As with Part B, record your answer by filling in the circle of the option.
4 Think about how the ideas in the answer options are different from each other.	

Part C

In this part of the test, you'll hear two different extracts. In each extract, you'll hear health professionals talking about aspects of their work.

For **questions 31–42**, choose the answer (**A**, **B** or **C**) which fits best according to what you hear. Complete your answers as you listen.

Now look at extract one.

Fill the circle in completely. Example: Ⓐ Ⓑ Ⓒ

Extract 1: Questions 31–36

You hear an interview with a nurse called Samira Heddon, who works for a charity that helps families affected by childhood continence issues.

You now have 90 seconds to read **questions 31–36**.

31 Samira explains that childhood incontinence remains a 'hidden problem' largely because

 Ⓐ parents are reluctant to seek assistance.

 Ⓑ children try to conceal symptoms from their parents.

 Ⓒ parents are unaware that problems occur outside the home.

Advice

31 Samira answers the question when she talks about 'families.' Listen to what she says about them and choose the option which matches what she says.

32 The charity was concerned to discover that the way continence issues were being dealt with in schools

- (A) generally failed to follow official guidance.
- (B) varied a great deal from one institution to another.
- (C) was usually based on the assumption that it was a family matter.

33 In selecting the main focus for their project, Samira's team was most influenced by

- (A) input from families with direct experience.
- (B) insights gained from the analysis of statistical data.
- (C) the volume of enquiries coming from the education sector.

34 Initially, the project group found it a challenge to decide how to

- (A) incorporate all the resources already in existence.
- (B) select the most appropriate age group to focus on.
- (C) ensure a broad range of perspectives was represented.

Advice

32 Samira says: 'What we found through our work was...' and then explains what they discovered, giving some examples. Which option matches what the charity found that 'didn't seem fair' to them?

33 All three options describe things that the team did, but which had the greatest influence? Listen to what Samira says about 'the aims' of the project.

34 Samira compares two things the team set out to do initially, saying one was 'straightforward' and the other was 'harder'. You're listening for what was harder to achieve.

35 What does Samira regard as the greatest strength of the document the group produced?

(A) the way it clarifies the role of the school

(B) the range of options it makes available tor teachers

(C) the personalised approach that it advocates for students

36 The example of Johan illustrates how the group's document can be used to help students

(A) to feel more confident about managing episodes of incontinence.

(B) to come to terms with different attitudes towards incontinence.

(C) to begin to understand the causes of their incontinence.

Now look at Extract 2.

Advice

35 Samira talks about three 'strengths' – or positive aspects – of the document. Listen for when she says: 'But for me, what really makes a difference is…'. This tells you that she's going to talk about the main strength.

36 Think about why Samira is telling us about Johan and the main idea in each option. Listen to the details of Johan's care plan. What has it helped him to do?

Extract 2: Questions 37–42

You hear a junior doctor called Ewen Garstang giving a presentation about different ways of dealing with large numbers of patients in an emergency department (ED).

You now have 90 seconds to read **questions 37–42**.

37 Ewen feels that the most serious effect of overcrowding in the ED relates to

(A) variations in the quality of care patients receive.

(B) feelings of discontent amongst both staff and patients.

(C) the long-term cost of patients receiving inadequate treatment.

38 Ewen would like to see all ED staff having some input in decisions about

(A) details of the physical layout of the space.

(B) different methods for managing the flow of patients.

(C) procedures for transferring patients to other departments.

Tip! In the presentation, the speaker indicates a change of sub-topic by taking a breath and introducing the new idea. Each question that you have to answer relates to one section of text.

Advice

37 The question is asking for the 'most serious effect'. Listen for the synonym 'crucially' which introduces this.

38 Ewen talks about all three things – but where does he think ED staff should have their input?

39 What drawback to traditional nurse triage does Ewen highlight?

(A) Patients aren't dealt with in an equal way.

(B) It leads to longer delays for the majority of patients.

(C) There's a risk of serious conditions going undetected.

40 What reservation about the idea of 'streaming' does Ewen voice?

(A) It can create confusion in the minds of patients.

(B) It relies on having staff with a wide range of skills.

(C) It creates an inflexible working pattern in the department.

41 What is Ewen's opinion of involving emergency doctors in triage?

(A) It may not be using their expertise to the best effect.

(B) It's an idea that should be tried more extensively.

(C) It can lead to increased levels of overcrowding.

42 What does Ewen suggest about point-of-care testing in the ED?

(A) It should be introduced more generally.

(B) It may be too expensive to be widely used.

(C) It needs to be trialled across the full range of tests.

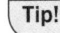 **Tip!** The punctuation tells you that 'streaming' is a term that you may not know.

Advice

39 The word 'drawback' means disadvantage. Ewen talks about both advantages and disadvantages of traditional nurse triage. Listen for when he changes from the positive to the negative aspects.

40 A 'reservation' is a doubt – so you're listening for why Ewen thinks streaming may not always be the best thing.

41 Ewen begins by explaining how this idea works in practice, then raises a doubt when he says: 'But you have to ask yourself whether ...'. Which of the three options matches Ewen's opinion?

42 Listen to everything Ewen says and decide which one best matches the point that he is making about it.

Task information

- The Speaking sub-test takes about 20 minutes in total and consists of two separate 5-minute role plays based on typical workplace consultations.

- Before the role plays begin, your identity and profession are checked, and there is a short warm-up conversation which is not assessed.

- You take the role of a doctor and an interlocutor a patient, client or carer. Role cards include details of the patient's condition and what you should cover.

- For each role play, you are given three minutes to prepare. You can make notes on the role card during the preparation time and ask any questions.

- You will not see the interlocutor's role card in the actual exam, but will do in this Trainer.

- The interlocutor will stop each role play conversation after five minutes.

- Your score is decided based on assessment criteria (see page 214).

Starting the role plays effectively

Each role card begins by explaining the context. Read this carefully so you can begin your consultation appropriately.

1  Read the background information on the role cards extracts below. Based on the information, make notes on what you might say to start the role play appropriately. Then listen to some samples and read the explanation in the Answer Key.

Tip! If you are unclear about what name to call the patient and/or carer, ask the interlocutor during the preparation.

A Setting: Doctor's Clinic
This 64-year-old with Type 2 diabetes is a regular patient of yours. You have just finished an examination of the patient's feet, during which you identified an infection.
- Give findings of your examination (superficial ulcer, slight purulence/warmth, etc.).

B Setting: Aged Care Facility
This 81-year-old patient has hypertension and rheumatoid arthritis. The Nursing Unit Manager has requested that you assess this patient because he/she has been experiencing problems when urinating. You are the on-call doctor and you are going to speak to this patient for the first time.
- Find out about patient's symptoms (e.g., onset, frequency, urgency, dysuria, incontinence, etc.).

Medical versus lay language

Use language suitable for speaking to a patient/carer during the role plays. Identify any medical terminology on the role card including bracketed information and decide how to express this appropriately in lay (everyday) language.

1  Listen to five pairs of extracts in which doctors are speaking to a patient. For each pair of extracts, write down which doctor (A or B) uses appropriate language for a patient/carer.

Tip! Identify language on the role card that might need to be explained in lay language during your planning time.

1 ....   2 ....   3 ....   4 ....   5 ....

2 Look at the following extract from a role card, in which the doctor is talking to a patient who has seasonal allergic rhinitis. Make notes on how you could transform the bracketed information into complete sentences for the patient.

- Outline treatment options (e.g., intranasal corticosteroids, antihistamines, decongestant sprays, etc.).
- Advise patient on lifestyle modifications (e.g., reducing exposure to triggers, use of pollen filter, showering/ changing clothes after being outside, etc.).

3  Listen to two doctors explaining the information in Exercise 2 to the patient. Decide which doctor (A or B) better transforms the information in brackets into meaningful sentences. Give reasons.

Active listening

Using active listening techniques when speaking to the patient in your role plays will facilitate patient participation and effective communication.

1 Complete the following definitions of active listening techniques by choosing the word(s) from the box.

> paraphrasing   clarification   back channelling   echoing

> **Tip!** Active listening often involves using these techniques in combination. The more variety you can show throughout the role plays, the better your Clinical Communication score should be.

1 .... is verbal encouragement given to the patient to show that you are paying attention, often through interjections like *uh-huh, OK, go on, really*?

2 .... is repeating the key words or last few spoken words by patient in the form of a question to encourage the patient to elaborate on what they are saying.

3 .... involves targeted questions to get more detail when the patient says something vague, or when you don't fully understand the patient.

4 .... means using putting into your own words what the patient has said, often simplifying it to a single idea. It allows you to verify your understanding, and encourages the patient to add anything that might have been missed.

2 Listen to four examples of active listening techniques described in Exercise 1 being demonstrated. For each one, write the technique being used.

1 ....   2 ....   3 ....   4 ....

Questioning techniques

Each role play includes information-gathering tasks (with verbs such as *Find out, Explore, Enquire about, Investigate, Ask*, etc.). Effective use of questioning is essential in getting the information you need.

1 Read the questioning techniques which follow. Choose an appropriate language example (a–e) and add it to the table.

Questioning technique	Language examples
1 Start the consultation with open questions to obtain a picture of the problem from the patient's perspective.	
2 Use closed questions when seeking a specific short answer or yes/no answer.	
3 Break up multi-questions so that each part can have its own separate answer.	
4 Use indirect questions to sound polite and unintrusive.	
5 When you've finished gathering information, summarise what the patient has told you. This helps to check the key details.	

a) Have you noticed any redness around the area? (Pause for patient's response) How about any swelling?

b) So, what can you tell me about the pain in your feet?

c) Do you cough during the night?

d) OK, so let me just check that I've got this right. You said…

e) Would you mind telling me how many cigarettes per day you smoke?

2  **Read the extract from a role card below. Listen to two different speakers taking the role of the doctor. Pay attention to the questioning techniques they use. Answer the questions below.**

You have just finished examining this 39-year-old patient, who has presented with lower back pain.
• Find out more about patient's back pain (e.g., onset, characteristics, severity, radiation, etc.).

1 Did Doctor A use effective or ineffective questioning techniques? Give reasons.

2 Did Doctor B use effective or ineffective questioning techniques? Give reasons.

3  **Listen again to the more effective doctor. Using the audio transcript, underline the examples of good questioning techniques. Add the good examples to the table in Exercise 1.**

Providing explanations

You will need to complete at least two information giving tasks during each role play. Information giving tasks begin with verbs such as *Explain, Educate, Inform, Give diagnosis of …*, etc.

1 Read the following explanation techniques. Put a tick (✓) for effective techniques when providing information to a patient/carer and a cross (✗) for ineffective techniques. Give reasons.

1 Find out how much the patient already knows about their own case.

2 Begin by outlining the topics you're going to cover in your explanation.

3 Speak without stopping until you've finished your explanation so that you can move on to the next task on the role card.

4 Pause periodically during your explanation.

5 Use 'signposting' language such as 'Firstly', 'In addition', 'On the other hand', 'As a consequence'.

6 Speak in the same tone of voice for the whole explanation.

2 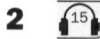  **Listen to two doctors, (A and B), explaining psoriasis. Pay attention to the explanation techniques they use. Answer the following questions.**

> **Tip!** You are not expected to have expert knowledge on the condition beyond the information provided on the card and will not be penalised if you make a factual error.

1 Did Doctor A use effective or ineffective explanation techniques? Give reasons.

2 Did Doctor B use effective or ineffective explanation techniques? Give reasons.

Action plan

Before the role plays begin

- Remember that before you start the role plays, your identity and profession will be checked, and you will be asked some questions about your professional background. This part of the test is not assessed.

During the role play preparation time

- Read the background information on the role card carefully.
- Identify whether or not you know the patient, and at what point in the consultation the role play starts. This will help you to start the role play appropriately.
- Try to identify the possible emotional needs of the patient and how urgent the situation is.
- Read each bulleted task carefully. Underline the verbs in each and consider how much time is needed for each action.
- Underline any medical terminology and decide how best to explain it the patient/carer.
- Plan how to structure your questions and explanations.
- Think about how you will use the information in brackets. Don't just read it as a list.

During each role play

- Try to relax – imagine you are speaking to a real patient or carer.
- Speak clearly throughout, emphasising key information and pausing frequently between ideas.
- Listen carefully to what the patient/carer says and personalise your responses to him/her.
- Maintain a patient-focused approach, particularly during any points of tension between you and the patient.
- You are not assessed on your medical knowledge, so don't worry if you make a factual error. You can even invent details if you need to.
- Don't rush. You are not penalised if you can't finish all the tasks.
- Don't add any tasks of your own. For example, don't take a history if you are not asked to.
- Remember it's OK to correct yourself if you make any mistakes.
- The interlocutor will indicate when each role play has finished so try to keep the conversation going until then.

Note that you are also provided with the interlocutor's role card here. In the actual exam, you will only see your own role card.

OET SAMPLE TEST

ROLEPLAYER CARD NO. 1   MEDICINE

SETTING	Doctor's Clinic
PATIENT	You are 64 years old and have high blood pressure and high cholesterol. The doctor has just finished assessing you using a cardiovascular risk calculator and is now going to talk to you about it.
TASK	• Say you didn't realise your health was so bad. • When asked, say you work long hours, so you don't have time to cook. You just eat a burger and fries for dinner most nights. You don't do any exercise. You drink a couple of glasses of wine every evening. • When asked, say you know that you need to eat healthier food and do more exercise, so you'll try to follow the doctor's advice. • Say you saw a news article about atorvastatin, and apparently, it can cause kidney failure. You don't want to take atorvastatin. • Say you're willing to try atorvastatin. You're relieved to hear that you'll be regularly monitored. • Say you'll come back for your follow-up appointment in eight weeks.

© Cambridge Boxhill Language Assessment (2022)   SAMPLE TEST

OET SAMPLE TEST

CANDIDATE CARD NO. 1   MEDICINE

SETTING	Doctor's Clinic
DOCTOR	This 64-year-old patient has hypertension (high blood pressure) and dyslipidaemia (high cholesterol). You have just completed a basic cardiovascular risk assessment of the patient and found him/her to be at high risk of cardiovascular disease.
TASK	• Give findings of your assessment (e.g., high risk of cardiovascular disease, 1 in 7 chance of heart attack/stroke within 5 years, etc.). • Find out about patient's lifestyle (e.g., diet, physical activity, alcohol intake, etc.). • Emphasise importance of lifestyle modification (e.g., healthy diet, increased physical activity, reduced alcohol intake, etc.). Explore patient's readiness to make lifestyle changes. • Recommend medication (e.g., atorvastatin to reduce blood cholesterol, proven to reduce risk of cardiovascular events, 1 tablet nightly, etc.). • Address patient's concerns about atorvastatin (e.g., low chance of serious/fatal side-effects, regular monitoring of patient, benefits outweigh risks, etc.). Establish patient's willingness to take atorvastatin. • Outline next steps (e.g., commencement of medication, follow-up appointment in eight weeks, cholesterol test, medication review, etc.).

© Cambridge Boxhill Language Assessment (2022)   SAMPLE TEST

OET SAMPLE TEST

ROLEPLAYER CARD NO. 2   MEDICINE

SETTING	Doctor's clinic
CARER	You've brought your two-year-old son to see the doctor. You think he has conjunctivitis. The doctor has just finished examining your son. Your son is now asleep.
TASK	• When asked, say your son started rubbing his eyes 3 days ago, and you noticed the eyes were red and watery. The eyelids stick together after he has been asleep. • When asked, say your son has had a cold for about a week. He's never had any problems with his eyes before and he doesn't take medication. • Say you think your son needs antibiotics as they will clear up the problem more quickly. • Say you understand why you can't have antibiotics. Say you'll use the compresses as advised. • Say you'll come back if your son's condition doesn't improve.

© Cambridge Boxhill Language Assessment (2022)   SAMPLE TEST

OET SAMPLE TEST

CANDIDATE CARD NO. 2   MEDICINE

SETTING	Doctor's Clinic
DOCTOR	This parent has brought in his/her two-year-old son with suspected conjunctivitis. You have just finished examining the child and found bilateral diffuse redness of the eyes with no foreign body. The child is now asleep.
TASK	• Find out about child's symptoms (e.g., onset, discharge, crusting, etc.). • Explore further details about child (e.g., any recent illnesses, history of eye conditions, medication use, etc.). • Confirm diagnosis of conjunctivitis (e.g., viral cause, highly contagious, spontaneous resolution in 1–2 weeks, etc). Advise on symptom relief (e.g., paracetamol if required, warm/cold compress several times daily, etc.). • Decline parent's request for antibiotics (e.g., ineffectiveness against viruses, contribution to antibiotic resistance, self-care sufficient, etc.). • Advise when follow-up appointment required (e.g., no improvement in three weeks).

© Cambridge Boxhill Language Assessment (2022)   SAMPLE TEST

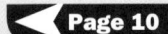 **Page 10**   *Task information*

Scanning with short answer questions.

The second set of questions for Part A focus on your ability to scan-read to locate specific information in the text in response to short questions.

1 Look at the examples of Reading Part A short answer questions and the box below which contains common foci for these questions. For each question, choose the type of information you are looking for.

> **Tip!** Because you will have completed questions 1–7 first, in the exam you should find it easier to decide which text is more likely to contain the answer/information you need.

the frequency of something   a method, procedure or treatment
a specific symptom   a quantity
associated conditions   an activity or action
a substance or material   the name of a drug or medication
a part of the body   a trigger or cause
a type of patient   when to do something

Question	Type of information needed
(8) What is the maximum dose per day of Mezavant XL?	
(9) Which medication can be broken up or dissolved in water?	
(10) Which habit have studies found helpful in preventing ulcerative colitis?	
(11) What is the best time of day to take Pentasa® retention enema?	

2 You may be able to scan the texts for key words from the question to help you locate the information you need. Look at the following questions. The focus of the question is underlined. Circle the word or words you need to scan the texts for.

> **Tip!** Answers should be short, normally one to three words, and should not repeat information given in the question.

  8 What is the <u>maximum dose per day</u> of Mezavant XL?

  9 Which <u>medication</u> can be <u>broken up or dissolved</u> in water?

 10 Which <u>habit</u> have studies found effective in <u>preventing</u> ulcerative colitis (UC)?

 11 What is the <u>best time of day</u> to take Pentasa retention enema?

3 Now look at Texts C and D. Skim-read them to decide in which text the answers to the questions in Exercises 1 and 2 are probably located. Then use the scan word(s) to find the answers to the questions.

Text C

Adult mesalazine dosage for treatment of acute attack of mild to moderate ulcerative colitis

	By mouth	By rectum
Asacol suppositories		0.75–1.5 g daily – divided doses, (final dose bedtime)
*Salofalk granules (place on tongue and wash down with water)	1.5–3 g mornings	
Pentasa retention enema		1 g daily (bedtime)
Asacol MR 800 mg tablets	2.4–4.8 g daily – divided doses.	
Mezavant XL	2.4 g daily increase if necessary to 4.8 g daily review after 8 weeks	
*Pentasa granules (place on tongue and wash down with water or orange juice)	Up to 4 g daily – single or divided doses	
Pentasa tablets (may be halved, quartered or dispersed in water.)	Up to 4 g once daily, alternatively up to 4 g daily in 2–3 divided doses.	

* Place on tongue and wash down with water – no chewing

Text D

Pathogenesis of Inflammatory Bowel Disease (IBD)
Pathogenesis reflects the complex interaction of multiple risk factors, including genetic and environmental components related to alterations in the gastrointestinal microbiota and immune system responses.
Key risk factors: genetic susceptibility, ethnicity, infection and environment (environmental factors linked to IBD correspond closely to Westernised diet, stress and activity levels)
Strongest links: smoking, gut microbiota, diet (high-fat, high-sugar) and medications (early and frequent exposure to antibiotics).

IBD and smoking have a complex relationship. An inverse association with UC (ulcerative colitis) exists and some research confirms that heavy smoking has a protective effect. Hospitalisation and colectomy rates, flare-ups and the need for oral steroids or immunosuppressants are all reported to be lower in smokers. However, the opposite is true for Crohn's Disease, as smokers are more likely to experience more severe symptoms and complications, such as strictures and fistulas.

Tip! In the actual exam you have a separate text booklet and question booklet. You write your answers in the question booklet.

Understanding the question focus in sentence completion tasks

Apply the same skills as for short answer questions (understanding the question focus, using scan words to search) for the sentence completion task. However, you may need to read more carefully as the question focus is less clear.

1 Look at the table below. For each gap, decide what type of information is needed. Use the common question foci box at the start of this section or your own ideas. The first one has been done for you as an example.

Incomplete sentence	Probable type of information needed	Probable word type
(15) Heavy use of .... in childhood is closely associated with IBD.	a substance or material / the name of a drug or medication	singular or plural noun
(16) .... of Pentasa and Salofalk granules is not recommended.		
(17) There is a strong connection between the lifestyle in .... cultures and IBD.		
(18) The minimum dose per day of Asacol suppositories is		

2 The incomplete sentence can also give you grammar clues to help you identify the type of word / phrase you need. Look at the questions in Exercise 1 again. Choose ideas from the box about the possible grammar of the answer you need and complete the third column. The first one has been done for you as an example.

> verb   number   verb + *-ing*   singular noun   plural noun

3 Look again at the incomplete sentences in Exercise 1 and the possible answer options for each below. Tick (✓) the correct answer (a or b) and choose an explanation (i–iv) for why the other option is an incorrect answer. The text that contains the answer is given in brackets to help you.

15 **a)** antiboitics   **b)** antibiotics   (Text D)

16 **a)** chewing of   **b)** chewing   (Text C)

17 **a)** Westernised   **b)** Western   (Text D)

18 **a)** 0.75   **b)** 0.75g / 0.75 grams   (Text C)

i)   the information is incomplete

ii)   spelling mistake

iii) the word used is not the same as in the text

iv) the answer repeats a word already in the sentence

> **Tip!** These are the four most common reasons for candidates losing marks.

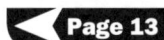 **Page 13**   *Action plan*

Pressure ulcers: Texts

Text A

Pressure ulcers, or bed sores, are any lesions caused by unrelieved pressure resulting in damage of the skin and/or underlying tissue. They usually occur over bony prominences as a result of pressure, or pressure with friction.

Patients who are particularly susceptible include those who are:

- aged >70
- confined to bed
- partially or completely immobile
- obese
- incontinent (urinary and faecal)
- malnourished
- have a circulation disorder
- have impaired sensation

Text B

Pressure ulcer stages

A staging system should be referred to in order to classify the degree of tissue damage observed. Darkly pigmented skin, casts or orthopedic devices can complicate and/or obstruct staging.

Description	Depth	Grade
Skin does not pale or lighten when pressed (darkly pigmented skin may turn blue / purple / violet) contrasting colour from periulcer skin • Warmth, pain, edema, hardness = possible indicators N.B. – use light finger palpitation for 10 seconds to determine whether skin pales or not	Shallow	1
Partial thickness loss of epidermis, or dermis or both Clinical presentation - abrasion, shallow crater, open/ruptured blister	Shallow	2
Partial thickness loss of epidermis, or dermis or both Clinical presentation - abrasion, shallow crater, open/ruptured blister	Deep	3
Full thickness tissue loss, with extensive destruction, tissue necrosis • Damage to bone, tendon and muscle • Slough, or dry, dead tissue may be present Often includes undermining and tunnelling	Deep	4

NB: Numerical identification of stages does not necessarily imply a progression in ulcer severity. For example, a stage 1 ulcer may have very little tissue damage, or it may have necrotic underlying tissue.

Cleansing and dressing

Wound cleansing	Wound dressing
All necrotic tissue, exudate and metabolic waste must be eliminated from the wound.	• necessary to maintain integrity of wound • should protect wound, be biocompatible and provide ideal hydration • condition of ulcer bed and desired dressing function determine type needed
Wound cleansing should take place initially and at each dressing stage. Remove all inflammatory foreign material, eg foreign bodies, residual topical agents, dressing residue.	**Use a dressing that will keep the ulcer bed continuously moist.** Wet-to-dry dressings are not considered continuously moist.
Do not use force when cleansing the ulcer with gauze, cloth or sponges. Coarse materials elicit more friction, trauma and infection.	**Use clinical judgement to select type of moist dressing.**
Do not use cleanser or antiseptic agents (eg. povidone iodine) as cytotoxic to normal tissue. Most cleansers must be diluted to maintain cell viability. Normal saline should be used for cleansing of most pressure ulcers.	**Dressings should keep periulcer skin dry and ulcer bed moist.** Skin is more likely to become infected when moist and must be therefore be protected from sources of excessive moisture (eg incontinence).
Apply sufficient irrigation pressure to enhance wound cleansing without traumatising wound bed. NB: Irrigation pressures that exceed 15psi may cause trauma and drive bacteria into the wound bed and tissue.	**Dressings should control exudate but not desiccate the ulcer bed.** Excessive exudate can macerate periulcer skin and should therefore be absorbed away from the ulcer bed.
	Eliminate wound dead space by loosely filling all cavities with dressing material. Cavities need to be filled to avoid abscesses. Overpacking may cause additional tissue damage.

Text D

Debridement

Moist, devitalised tissue supports the growth of pathological organisms. Therefore, eliminating such tissue favourably alters the healing environment of a wound. Debridement methods should be selected according to the patient's condition and goals. Urgent clinical need for drainage or removal of devitalised tissue, such as advancing cellulitis or sepsis calls for urgent debridement, and the sharp method should be used.

Debridement methods:

Sharp: used to remove thick, adherent eschar and devitalised tissue in larger, more serious ulcers, with a sharp instrument. Often done at the bedside, or in an operating theatre for extensive wounds.

Mechanical: can be used as the sole form or an initial form, while the patient is being prepared for surgery. Wet-to-dry dressings adhere to devitalised tissue, when dry this is removed along with dressing.

Enzymatic: Suitable for patients who cannot tolerate surgery, those in long-term care or whose ulcer is not infected. Involves topical application of debriding agents to devitalised tissues on the wound surface.

The newer fluorinated derivatives (ciprofloxacin and ofloxacin) have been successfully used to treat complicated skin and soft tissue infections such as abscesses, cellulitis, and infected pressure ulcers caused by multi-resistant Gram-negative bacteria. Ciprofloxacin is best administered orally, as this method induces rapid absorption.

Part A

TIME: 15 minutes

- Look at the four texts, **A–D**, in the separate **Text Booklet** that precedes the questions.

- For each question, **1–20**, look through the texts, **A–D**, to find the relevant information.

- Write your answers on the spaces provided in this **Question Paper**.

- Answer all the questions within the 15-minute time limit.

- Your answers should **only** be taken from texts **A–D** and must be correctly spelt.

Pressure Ulcers: Questions

Questions 1–7

For each question, **1–7**, decide which text (**A**, **B**, **C** or **D**) the information comes from. You may use any letter more than once.

In which text can you find information about

1	how to categorise a pressure ulcer?	_____
2	when dead tissue should be removed without delay?	_____
3	what to consider when deciding how to cover a pressure ulcer?	_____
4	a method for testing whether skin colour fades under pressure?	_____
5	what a pressure ulcer is?	_____
6	people who are most at risk of developing pressure ulcers?	_____
7	how to safely disinfect a wound?	_____

Advice

1 Which text gives information on classification of ulcers?

2 Which text's title matches with the idea here?

3 Which text gives information on dressings?

4 Which text refers a lot to skin colour?

5 You are looking for a definition.

6 Look for a synonym of 'at risk of' and a description of patients.

7 The key words here is 'wound'. Two text mention it a lot, but only one mentions 'disinfecting' though it uses a different word.

Questions 8–13

Answer each of the questions, **8–13**, with a word or short phrase from one of the texts. Each answer may include words, numbers or both.

8 How long should you apply pressure for to check whether the skin lightens?

_____

9 Which solution should usually be used to clean a wound?

_____

10 Where on the body is a pressure ulcer most likely to appear?

_____

Advice

8 Look in text B for this.

9 A solution is a type of liquid.

10 Look in a text that gives a definition of pressure ulcers.

11 Which type of dressing is not recommended for pressure ulcers?

_____

12 What can occur if a wound is left with no packing?

_____

13 What is the most appropriate way to give ciprofloxacin when treating a pressure ulcer?

_____

Advice

11 _Only one text talks extensively about dressings so scan it for one that is not suitable and the reason why ._

12 _Filling is a synonym for packing here, so scan for that._

13 _The key word here is 'ciprofloxacin'. Look for a word on how to administer it._

Questions 14–20

Complete each of the sentences, **14–20**, with a word or short phrase from one of the texts. Each answer may include words, numbers or both.

14 When removing dead tissue from extensive wounds the

_____ method should be used.

15 The tissue surrounding the wound can become macerated if

_____ is not controlled by the dressing.

16 When cleaning an ulcer, water pressure needs to be less than

_____ .

17 A deep ulcer with significant deterioration of the flesh is classified as grade

_____ .

18 The development of _____ _____ is encouraged by dead tissue.

19 A category 1 ulcer may be a different

_____ to the surrounding area.

20 Patients over the age of _____ are more prone to pressure ulcers.

Advice

14 _Look in a text that focuses on removing dead tissue._

15 _Look in a text about dressings for mention or maceration._

16 _Look for a number and abbreviation related to pressure._

17 _Look in the text that focuses on grading ulcers._

18 _You need a two-word terms here._

19 _One of the texts describes different ways to classify ulcers but doesn't use the word 'category'._

20 _The answer is a number, but the text uses a synonym for 'prone to' before the answer._

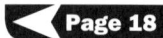 **Page 18**   *Task information*

Gist questions

Gist reading questions ask you to determine what the text is mostly about. Sometimes gist and the main idea are the same, but generally speaking, gist is the subject matter of a text whereas the main idea is what the writer wants to communicate about the subject matter.

1   Look at the sample Part B text (guidelines) and two possible Part B question stems below (without answer options) that you could be asked about it. Decide which question is asking for the gist (G) and which the purpose (D) of the text.

Malaria

Malaria prophylaxis is not absolute, and breakthrough infection can occur with any of the recommended drugs. Travellers to affected areas should be made aware that additional defensive measures, such as wearing suitable clothing after sunset, sleeping in well-sealed rooms and use of mosquito bed nets and insect repellent, are essential.

When applied correctly, a 50% DEET-based repellent is the gold standard. Incorrect use can result in irritation, redness and swelling of the skin and eyes. Ingestion may result in vomiting, nausea and, in extreme case, seizures. However, it is safe and effective for children over 2 months of age and can also be used during pregnancy and breast-feeding provided hands and breast tissue are cleaned thoroughly before handling infants. When sunscreen is also required, DEET should be applied after using a sunscreen with an SPF (sun protection factor) of 30–50.

---

1   This guideline about malaria gives information about
2   This guideline about malaria was written to advise staff that

2   Look at question 1 again. Read the text. What aspect of malaria do you think it is focusing on? Write down your ideas.

3   Now look at the answer options for question 1. The key words in the options have been underlined. Which option best matches your ideas in Exercise 2 and summarises the overall message?
   A some common complications of the disease.
   B medications that can be taken to treat the disease.
   C different methods of protection against the disease.

Tip! Gist questions require a global understanding of the text, so skimming is a useful reading skill here as you don't need to understand every word, just the topic and direction of the text.

Purpose questions

Some Part B questions ask you to decide the purpose of a text – what the text is telling the relevant medical professional(s) to do, know or remember in certain contexts or circumstances.

1 Answer options for 'purpose' questions often begin with verbs that give a specific action or function that reflects the purpose of the text. Look at the box below which contains verbs that may begin answer options. Choose the verb whose meaning/function best matches the meaning/function of the sentences. The first one has been done for you.

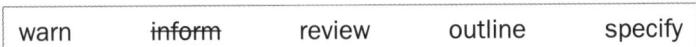

| warn | ~~inform~~ | review | outline | specify |

1 Any incidents should be reported immediately to the senior nurse on duty.   *inform*

2 Before discharge, check again with the patient that they understand how to take all prescribed medicines.

3 It is essential to indicate the exact quantity of the specimen and the time it was taken.

4 Make patients aware that ginkgo boloba interferes with warfarin and therefore raises the risk of thrombosis.

Tip! Other common function verbs for purpose questions include recommend, explain, give guidance on, and help.

5 It's advisable at this stage to give an overview of what the treatment options are, including potential side effects, so that the patient can make an informed choice.

2 Purpose questions often focus on language in the text that expresses obligation, advice, and recommendation. Look at these sentences that could come from Part B texts. Decide if the underlined sections express obligation (O), recommendation (R), or prohibition (P).

1 <u>Under no circumstances should</u> the procedure go ahead without all the relevant consent forms being signed.

2 All employees <u>are required to</u> attend an informal meeting.

3 <u>Users should be provided with</u> dietary and drug interaction advice before discharge.

3 Now read the sample Part B text (guidelines) and the 'purpose' question that follows. Think about who the text is for and what it is asking them to do. Then choose the correct answer.

> ### Guidelines on treatment of anxiety disorders
>
> Pharmacological treatment of anxiety disorders should only be offered for severe and persistent symptoms which result in occupational and social disability. The condition and treatment options must be discussed fully and written information provided. It is vital that patients be made aware of the likely duration of treatment, the importance of compliance and that antidepressants have a delayed onset period of a minimum of two weeks. Explain and clarify the regimen and check the patient understands the importance of compliance. Responses should be evaluated and noted at each review and the treatment adjusted if deemed necessary. Note that benzodiazepines and antipsychotics are not suitable for people with anxiety disorders.

Tip! Words or ideas from the incorrect answer options may be mentioned in the text. However, you need to check that the ideas in the options fully match what the text says AND answer the question.

The purpose of this guideline on pharmacological treatment of anxiety disorders is to

A warn about the side effects of certain types of medication.

B outline the responsibilities of the doctor when prescribing medication.

C specify the procedure to be followed if patients fail to respond to medication.

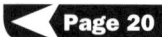 **Page 20** *Action plan*

Part B

In this part of the test, there are six short extracts relating to the work of health professionals. For **questions 1–6**, choose the answer (**A**, **B** or **C**) which you think fits best according to the text.

Fill the circle in completely. Example:

Ⓐ
Ⓑ
Ⓒ

---

1 What point do the guidelines make about allocating powered wheelchairs?

  Ⓐ Patients with progressive conditions should be prioritised.

  Ⓑ Extra care should be taken when assessing their suitability for a child.

  Ⓒ Every effort should be made to offer them to the widest possible range of users.

Wheelchair selection guidelines

Mechanisms in wheelchairs which are used to provide seat tilt, seat lift and backrest recline functions can pose an entrapment threat, in particular to fingers, toes and especially to inquisitive children. Trapping points can also be created when adjustable components such as reclining backrests are moved relative to fixed components such as armrests. During the evaluation process, consideration should be given to the user's physical abilities (e.g. eyesight and postural control) and the intended setting for the wheelchair, along with the manufacturer's guidance, to reduce trapping hazards. People who are visually impaired or who have severe epilepsy may be unable to use powered wheelchairs safely. However, the benefits, specific situation, diagnosis and prognosis should be taken into account, so that end users, who could in fact operate the powered wheelchair safely, are not denied.

> **Advice**
>
> *1 Focus on the part of the text that discusses **powered** wheelchairs.*

2 The memo about animal euthanasia advises veterinary surgeons on

   (A) how to recognise when an owner is neglectful.

   (B) how best to support owners after the procedure.

   (C) what to do if owners' wishes conflict with their opinion.

Advice

2 The text advises veterinary surgeons on what to do or consider before deciding if euthanasia is appropriate which immediately rules out one option.

3 Consider the verbs at the beginning of each answer option carefully.

Memo for veterinary surgeons: Euthanasia

The primary purpose of euthanasia is to relieve the suffering of an animal. Before a decision is made, many factors should be assessed, including extent and nature of the disease or injuries, prognosis and potential quality of life after treatment, likelihood of successful treatment, animal's age and health status or even the owner is able to pay for private treatment.

On occasion, veterinary surgeons may need to make difficult decisions. For example, they may receive a request for the destruction of an animal which, in their clinical and professional judgement, is unnecessary, as there are no health or welfare reasons. Conversely, an owner may wish to keep an animal alive in circumstances where euthanasia would be the kindest course of action. In such cases, the extreme sensitivity of the situation should be recognised, and sympathetic efforts made to recommend alternative sources of advice, such as a second veterinary opinion.

---

3 The memo states that patients presenting with influenza symptoms should be

   (A) started on medication before the illness is confirmed.

   (B) placed in isolation to protect other patients.

   (C) examined for other high-risk conditions.

Memo: To all family doctors – influenza diagnosis

This is a reminder that influenza must be considered in patients presenting with compatible symptoms and verified rapidly by requesting appropriate laboratory investigations. It is equally important that empirical antiviral therapy is commenced rapidly, before influenza is identified, as delays are associated with increased mortality.

Seasonal influenza: Patients with severe, complicated influenza often require admission to critical care units at the time of hospitalisation or soon after admission. Influenza may be missed as a potential diagnosis in individuals who have travelled recently, have unexplained severe, acute respiratory infections or out-of-season, atypical or extra-pulmonary presentations. In addition to consequences for the infected individual, failure to consider influenza and implement appropriate infection prevention and control measures may increase the risk of in-hospital transmission and outbreaks within critical care.

---

4   The guideline about the use of gloves informs the reader about

   (A)   when they should be worn.

   (B)   why regional protocols vary.

   (C)   how to take them off safely.

Advice

4 In the answer options, consider the question words 'how' (which method) 'when' (what times/occasions) and 'why' (for what reasons)? The text only focuses on one of these.

5 Locate the section of text which discusses antipsychotics. Look at how this section is organised. Disadvantages are discussed first, followed by when prescription may be acceptable.

Guideline for nurses: Use of sterile and non-sterile gloves

Gloves are not a substitute for hand hygiene and should only be used when appropriate. Their prolonged and unnecessary use may cause adverse reactions, skin sensitivity and cross-contamination of the patient environment. Routine use is expected when anticipating contact with bodily fluids or chemical hazards and when handling sharps or contaminated devices. It may also be required as part of local policy for managing transmission-based precautions (droplet, airborne or contact).

When undertaking an aseptic non-touch technique, sterile or non-sterile gloves should be selected in line with procedure and local policy. Any cuts or abrasions should be covered using a waterproof dressing before putting gloves on and hands must be thoroughly decontaminated after removal.

They are a single use item and must therefore be disposed of immediately after the care activity for which they have been worn.

---

5   What does the guideline say about prescribing antipsychotics to patients with dementia?

   (A)   It is only appropriate if used for a clearly defined period of time.

   (B)   It is worth considering as long as a patient has no comorbidities.

   (C)   It can be done if circumstances are so severe that there is no alternative.

Prescribing guidelines: Alzheimer's

Although antipsychotics are sometimes prescribed for behavioural and psychological symptoms of dementia, they produce limited benefits and are associated with an increased risk of stroke and mortality, as well as other serious adverse events such as sedation and accelerated cognitive decline. However, in cases of dementia associated with extreme disturbance that require urgent treatment, for example, if violence, aggression or severe agitation are present, an antipsychotic drug or a benzodiazepine may be given as a last resort.

Before commencing, the benefits and harms should be discussed with the patient, family members and carers, as appropriate. The antipsychotic should be used at the lowest dose for the shortest possible time. It should be stopped if it is not helping or is no longer needed.

---

6 What does the guideline say is true in the majority of cases of out-toeing?

(A) Both feet are affected to similar degree.

(B) The problem will resolve naturally over time.

(C) It is not possible to identify the underlying cause.

Advice

6 *Look for a synonym for 'the majority of cases'.*

Guidance: Out-toeing in young children

Out-toeing is when the toes point in an outwards direction when walking and is most commonly seen in early walkers. Although it may also be associated with 'knock knees' and 'flatfoot', restricted internal rotation of the hip is the most common cause. Serious underlying causes, such as slipped upper femoral epiphysis, should be excluded before parents can be reassured that in most instances, the issue corrects itself as the child grows and intervention is not usually necessary.

A thorough observation of the gait should be carried out, then the child placed in prone position for an examination of range of motion in the internal and external hip, foot posture and thigh-foot angle, which should not exceed 30–40 degrees. Children who are showing signs of asymmetrical deformity, functional difficulties or progression of out-toeing should be referred immediately.

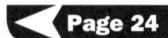 **Page 24**   *Task information*

Lexis questions

Lexis questions ask you to explain the use of a word or phrase in the text (highlighted in bold and underlined). These questions are not testing your vocabulary knowledge, but rather your ability to understand meaning in the context of the text.

1   Look at the sixth paragraph below, which is the final paragraph from the TB text we saw in Test 1 Training. Look at the word and phrase underlined and in bold. For each, choose the option (a or b) which best fits the meaning in the context of the paragraph.

> The discoveries in Dja'de el'Mughara and Tell Aswad are incredibly important. Finding evidence of TB in people who died 10,000 years ago challenges the long-held belief about its origins and has led to some **(1) wrangling** among the medical research community. But researchers now generally believe that TB in humans did not originate from cattle domestication and that the disease has been afflicting our ancestors for far longer than we imagined. This evidence could prove to be **(2) the piece of the jigsaw** that revolutionises our understanding and approach to this deadly disease which claims the lives of at least 1.7 million people every year.

   1   a) disagreement
        b) negotiation
   2   a) the puzzle
        b) the solution

2   Now look at the fourth and fifth paragraphs from the TB text and the sample 'lexis' question stem (without answer options). Focus on the bold and underlined phrase and the text that follows it. What does it tell us about Oussama Baker and his colleagues examining bodies from Dja'de el'Mughara?

> However, the study of ancient diseases needn't rely solely on this sort of evidence. In recent years, advances in genetics mean palaeopathologists can also use ancient and modern DNA to reconstruct the evolution of pathogens. And there is some genetic evidence suggesting that Kappelman may have been on to something. In 2002, a study led by Roland Brosch at the Pasteur Institute in Paris concluded that M. tuberculosis is older in origin than M. bovis, suggesting it evolved in humans before cattle domestication.

> Researchers then started to look for evidence in fossils in a site called Dja'de el'Mughara, on the western bank of the Euphrates river, which was first inhabited by humans around 11,300 years ago. People practised proto-agriculture there from the beginning, and the site also has the earliest known evidence of domestication of a cow-like animal, the now-extinct auroch, dating from around 10,000 years ago. **With that information in mind**, Oussama Baker at EPHE in Paris and his colleagues carefully examined 130 bodies from the site. They found signs of TB infection in 10 bodies dating to between 8000 and 10,000 years ago. Seven of these people lived during the transition to cattle domestication. However, the most ancient, which include an infant who died around the age of 1, predate domestication. Analysis of ancient DNA confirmed the diagnosis. What's more, the team found another skeleton with evidence of TB at a Syrian site called Tell Aswad. The skeleton belonged to a young adult and dates to between 7600 and 8200 years ago, which again precedes cattle domestication there.

The phrase '**with that information in mind**' in the fifth paragraph suggests that Oussama Baker

Tip! Lexis questions may focus on common words or phrases but you need to think carefully about what these mean in the specific context of the text.

3 Now look at the answer options for the question in Exercise 2 and choose the correct answer.
   A already knew that researchers had found evidence of TB in bodies at the site.
   B was aware that the site was suitable for following up the work of earlier researchers.
   C was reminded that remains found at the site were of an animal which is now extinct.
   D remembered work he had done in a previous location when he started working at the site.

'Purpose of an example' questions

Longer academic texts often include examples related to the topic, such as a case study, similar research or projects, in order to help the writer demonstrate a point they are making. Think carefully about what the writer is trying to communicate by means of the example and choose the answer option which best explains this.

1 Look again at the fifth paragraph and at the sample question stem (without answer options). Underline in the text where the finding at Tell Aswad is mentioned. Then read the sentences around it and decide why you think it was mentioned.

Researchers then started to look for evidence in fossils in a site called Dja'de el'Mughara, on the western bank of the Euphrates river, which was first inhabited by humans around 11,300 years ago. People practised proto-agriculture there from the beginning, and the site also has the earliest known evidence of domestication of a cow-like animal, the now-extinct auroch, dating from around 10,000 years ago. With that in mind, Oussama Baker at EPHE in Paris and his colleagues carefully examined 130 bodies from the site. They found signs of TB infection in 10 bodies dating to between 8000 and 10,000 years ago. Seven of these people lived during the transition to cattle domestication. However, the most ancient, which include an infant who died around the age of 1, predate domestication. Analysis of ancient DNA confirmed the diagnosis. What's more, the team found another skeleton with evidence of TB at a Syrian site called Tell Aswad. The skeleton belonged to a young adult and dates to between 7600 and 8200 years ago, which precedes cattle domestication there.

The writer refers to a skeleton found at a site called Tell Aswad in order to

Tip! The purpose of the example is often shown by the text that follows the example, but in this case the purpose is revealed in the preceding and subsequent sentences.

2 Now look at the answer options and decide which one best matches your ideas in Exercise 1.
   A exemplify the physical features that indicate the presence of TB.
   B suggest that TB affected people as well as animals in early societies.
   C provide further evidence that cattle couldn't pass TB to humans.
   D support the idea that TB was widespread among humans at an early date.

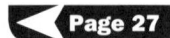

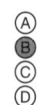

◄ **Page 27** *Action plan*

Part C

In this part of the test, there are two texts about different aspects of healthcare. For **questions 7–22**, choose the answer (**A**, **B**, **C** or **D**) which you think fits best according to the text.

Fill the circle in completely. Example:

Ⓐ
Ⓑ
Ⓒ
Ⓓ

Text 1: Measles vaccine hesitancy

Measles is a highly contagious and potentially fatal disease caused by a paramyxovirus. It infects the respiratory tract and spreads throughout the body, causing a blotchy red-brown rash and high fever, as well as complications including encephalitis, seizures and brain damage. A safe and effective vaccine was introduced in 1963, yet despite the fact that measles is now preventable, there has been a rapid escalation in global epidemics, with cases increasing tenfold in Africa since 2006 and fourfold in Europe since 2017. In 2018, almost ten million cases and more than 140,000 deaths were reported, mostly amongst children under the age of five. The World Health Organisation (WHO) claims that 'all cases are because people who should have been vaccinated were not', underlining the need to invest in education, immunisation and quality health care as a right for all.

In developing countries, weak healthcare systems may be partly to blame for low vaccination rates. However, this is not the case in developed countries, where anti-vaccine sentiment has had a more substantial impact. In the UK, measles, mumps and rubella (MMR) coverage is now well below the recommended 95% to ensure effective herd immunity and as a result it has lost its WHO measles elimination status. Analysis of vaccine hesitancy and falling uptake has highlighted the role of social media activism and pseudoscience in incorrectly portraying vaccination as harmful, unproven and responsible for the rise in illness or disorders such as autism. Individual liberty and parents' right to choose are common reasons given for vaccine refusal. Right wing populism, with its suspicion of authority, intellectuals and professionals is also thought to have played a role.

However, the majority of parents do not have the benefit of understanding the principles of toxicology, immunology, epidemiology or biostatistics and so they are understandably sceptical. After all, we do not allow children to put toxins in their mouth, so for many the idea of permitting a stranger to inject their young child with a fatal disease really **goes against the grain**. Furthermore, many object for religious or philosophical reasons. If we are serious about increasing protection levels, we need to fully understand the rationale behind vaccine refusal and listen more sympathetically to those who oppose it. Only then can we work out how to persuade them to have the vaccination.

One controversial idea that has been proposed in the UK is compulsory vaccination for children, although the practicalities and repercussions of implementing such an ambitious plan remain unclear. The WHO leaves individual countries to decide their own way of ensuring high rates and makes no recommendation for or against mandating. Some countries make vaccination a condition for attending school and others use the threat of withholding benefits, such as social security payments. Furthermore, studies examining Europe's different governmental approaches did not point to a single best one and highlighted the likelihood of unwelcome outcomes of compulsion, including a lack of proper education for some, as a significant proportion of parents will not be persuaded to change their mind when faced with obligation.

Emerging research highlights the importance of vaccination against measles. Michael Mina pioneered a study at Harvard University and discovered that the disease has a devastating effect on the immune system, making it far more lethal than we realised. He coined the term 'immune amnesia' for the phenomenon he uncovered. Experts suspect that it may be a catalyst for many deaths from other illnesses, that would otherwise not have been contracted. During childhood, as we are infected with diseases or are vaccinated against them, we accumulate specialised immune cells, each of which has learned to produce antibodies to attack one particular part of a pathogen. Two major studies of members of the Dutch Orthodox church, which rejects vaccination, discovered that the measles virus kills up to 73% of these cells. Immunity is gradually regained as they are re-exposed, but in the meantime people remain susceptible to serious complications of those infections. In the light of this finding, Mina believes that patients recovering from measles would benefit hugely from a round of booster shots of all previous routine vaccines, as the long-term consequences that stem from increased susceptibility are potentially devastating.

All of the effects observed in this study occurred in previously healthy children. Because measles is known to hit malnourished children much harder, the degree of immune amnesia and its effects could be even more severe in less healthy populations. Ensuring widespread vaccination would not only help prevent the deaths directly attributed to measles but could also avert potentially hundreds of thousands of additional deaths attributable to the lasting damage to the immune system. '**This** drives home the importance of understanding and preventing the long-term effects of measles, including stealth effects that have flown under the radar of doctors and parents,' said Mina. 'The symptoms of measles itself may be the tip of the iceberg.'

Text 1: Questions 7–14

7   In the first paragraph, the writer's purpose is to explain why

   (A)   measles symptoms are easily mistaken for those of other diseases.

   (B)   there has been a recent rise in the number of measles cases.

   (C)   solving the problem of measles in Africa will not be easy.

   (D)   the death rate for measles in the under 5s is increasing.

Advice

7 This question is essentially asking for the purpose or main idea of the first paragraph.

8 Find the section of text which indicates that fewer people are being vaccinated. The text which follows offers explanations and only one answer option accurately represents them.

9 The answer is given before the phrase appears in the text.

10 The answer is in the same paragraph as the previous question but comes after the phrase.

8   In the second paragraph, one reason the writer gives for refusal of the measles vaccination is

   (A)   infrequent encounters of the disease in day to day life.

   (B)   a lack of understanding of the severity of the disease.

   (C)   fear of impairments it has been said to cause.

   (D)   insufficient guidance from experts.

9   The writer uses the phrase '**goes against the grain**' to emphasise his feeling that

   (A)   fear of vaccines is not necessarily irrational.

   (B)   children's needs must be put before parents'.

   (C)   improving science education should be a priority.

   (D)   it's hard to make people do what is expected of them.

10   What approach to improving vaccine take-up does the writer advocate in the third paragraph?

   (A)   making vaccination centres more accessible and family-friendly

   (B)   raising awareness of the potential impact of childhood disease

   (C)   offering parents a simple explanation of how vaccines work

   (D)   considering the perspective of those who have concerns

11 What problem with compulsory vaccination does the writer identify in the fourth paragraph?

(A) There is no united international approach.

(B) It could lead to significant social inequalities.

(C) Most countries lack the public funding to enforce it.

(D) It would require countries to change their welfare systems.

12 What do we learn from the fifth paragraph about the research that Michael Mina carried out?

(A) It confirmed a theory that had already been put forward.

(B) There are a number of different ways to interpret the data.

(C) It has helped persuade some populations to get vaccinated.

(D) There is a way to deal with the additional risks it revealed.

13 In the final paragraph, '**This**' refers to the fact that measles vaccination programmes

(A) require more thorough research in developing countries.

(B) are likely to be more straightforward in wealthy countries.

(C) may have a more profound impact than originally intended.

(D) generate valuable data that can be applied to other diseases.

14 What is Mina doing in the quotation at the end of the final paragraph?

(A) emphasising the need to recognise the true impact measles can have

(B) reinforcing his concerns about the direction of future measles research

(C) demonstrating the support he feels for those who treat measles patients

(D) expressing the pride he feels that his measles research has been so influential

Advice

11 Two of the answer options are true, but only one is cited as an 'unwelcome outcome'.

12 Consider the verbs in each option ('put forward', 'interpret', 'persuade' and 'deal with'. Which of these ideas is best summarised in the text?

13 You are looking for something that the studies revealed or uncovered about measles.

14 Focus on the first three words of each option.

Text 2: Helminth therapy

Intestinal worms, or helminths, are thought to inhabit at least 2 billion people worldwide. Last year, Alex Loukas deliberately joined their ranks by introducing larvae of the parasitic New World hookworm into his forearm. Loukas, a researcher at James Cook University in Australia, has concluded through his work that despite their reputation, infection with helminths isn't always harmful. In fact, he argues that there could be some unique benefits to controlled, low-level infection with certain species. As an advocate for exploring this as a potential therapy, Loukas realised he had to undergo it himself.

Self-infection as practised by Loukas isn't uncommon among people with severe inflammatory diseases. Researchers at the University of California identified one such case: a 35-year-old man, diagnosed with ulcerative colitis, who had swallowed whipworm eggs. Remarkably, they found that his previously inflamed colon showed less damage a year on. This improvement was not a one-off either: after experiencing worsening symptoms alongside declining helminth egg numbers, the man re-infected himself and experienced the same calming of symptoms. Moreover, while his gut had contained T-helper cells producing an inflammatory cytokine just prior to his infection, it subsequently began producing a cytokine involved in repairing the gut wall – as if the worms were restoring the mucosal barrier.

Often referred to as immunoregulators, helminths secrete and excrete vast quantities of proteins and other molecules that influence the activity of the host's immune system. It's a survival strategy born of necessity for a large parasite which can survive for years in a single gut and which, unlike a bacterium or virus, can't out-multiply its host's defenses. Helminths have been co-evolving with humans for our entire history. Until improved hygiene and healthcare began to wipe out worm infections in industrialized countries, "the whole human population would have had these parasites for most of their life," says immunologist Rick Maizels.

This intimate biological relationship forms the basis for the argument that helminths are vital for keeping harmful immune responses in check – and that their absence might account for some of the observed increases in autoimmune and inflammatory disorders, such as allergies. It's a controversial theory. Parasitic diseases expert Peter Hotez has questioned whether the associations are causal, noting how research has found that many helminths can exacerbate or even promote inflammatory conditions. But although Loukas, Maizels, and others agree that some helminth infections can be dangerous, they speculate that manipulation of the immune system by more benign species may limit harmful immune responses.

Previous attempts to convert this line of thinking into therapies for immune-related conditions have had mixed success. In the early 2000s, clinical trials of helminth infection as a treatment for conditions including Crohn's disease, celiac disease, and asthma generally produced unimpressive results. A trial of celiac patients published recently, for example, failed to find a positive impact of hookworm infection on gluten tolerance, although some helminth-positive participants did report improved well-being and quality of life. However, it is worth noting, as Loukas himself did, that the researchers had had trouble establishing stable infections in some participants, perhaps because the worms fared badly on the flight to the New Zealand trial site. An earlier trial led by the same group had suggested a beneficial effect of worm infection on gluten tolerance, but wasn't placebo-controlled.

The complexity of worm-host interactions makes it hard to know whether negative trial results prove that a helminth therapy is ineffective, or just that it only helps specific patients. Proponents of helminth therapy are now approaching **this** issue from a different angle, placing stronger emphasis on understanding the mechanisms underlying host/helminth interactions. They view both the worm and the individual compounds it secretes as potential therapeutics.

One approach to helminth-based therapy may be to **remove the worm**, a multicellular animal with its own lifecycle and behavior **from the equation** altogether. Studies of secretions and excretions from the dog hookworm have identified 315 different proteins present. Others have studied the, secretions of Heligmosomoides polygyrus, an intestinal rodent parasite, and discovered that one, the enzyme glutamate dehydrogenase, inhibited immune reactions. Intranasal treatment with this molecule supressed allergic airway inflammation in mice, and could form the basis of treatment for asthma-related conditions.

Another way could be to learn more about the body's responses to the presence of helminths. Helminths are often associated with changes in the composition of bacterial species in the gut – the gut microbiota – something that is increasingly linked to disease risk and outcomes irrespective of infection by helminths and the like. Circumstantial evidence for this comes from findings that worm-infected people have different microbiomes than uninfected people. One study found that helminth infection can completely remodel the gut microbiota in mice, for example. And in a clinical trial of celiac patients, Loukas reported that experimental infection led to a small but statistically significant increase in the number of gut bacteria species. This underlines the complexity of the body's biological community – and the amount there is to learn before worms or their derivatives can be used therapeutically

Text 2: Questions 15–22

15   What is the writer doing in the first paragraph?

(A)   describing the medical advantages of helminth infection

(B)   explaining the motivation behind an experiment with helminths

(C)   introducing an innovative use of helminths in healthcare

(D)   identifying varieties of helminths that have a medical application

16   What aspect of helminth therapy is exemplified by the man mentioned in the second paragraph?

(A)   the speed at which it can take effect on patients

(B)   the relative effectiveness of it as a treatment

(C)   the type of patient who has found it helpful

(D)   the frequency with which certain patients use it

17   In the third paragraph, the writer says that the impact of helminths on an individual

(A)   depends on the ability of that person's immune system to resist them.

(B)   is partly due to their need to overcome the human body's natural reaction to parasites.

(C)   has been strengthened through their long association with humans.

(D)   may have been intensified by lifestyle changes in developed countries.

18   In the fourth paragraph, the writer's reference to Hotez, Loukas and Maizels illustrates disagreements over

(A)   the way that helminth therapy should be applied to patients.

(B)   the potential benefits that helminth therapy could offer.

(C)   the link between helminths and a recent rise in certain medical conditions.

(D)   the safety risks of using helminths to treat certain medical conditions

Advice

15 The writer's focus here is Alex Loukas. What did he do and why?

16 Find the condition the man in the example suffered from. How it this related to the first sentence of the paragraph?

17 Identify what helminths do to the body and why?

18 Locas and Maizels agree with in part with Hotez but not on one aspect. Which?

19 In the fifth paragraph, what does the writer suggest about both of the two clinical trials of helminth therapy?

(A) There were certain doubts about their reliability.

(B) They relied too much on participants' anecdotal evidence.

(C) There were too few subjects for them to reach definite conclusions.

(D) They demonstrated the difficulties in administering such treatments.

20 In the sixth paragraph, what does the word **this** refer to?

(A) support for the use of helminth therapy

(B) evaluating the impact of helminths on specific patients

(C) interpreting the outcomes of helminth therapy trials

(D) understanding the relationship between helminths and their host

21 The reference to **removing the worm... from the equation** suggests that the helminths may be

(A) distorting some of the clinical research results.

(B) too unpredictable in its activities for any effective study.

(C) responsible for causing excessive physical damage to their hosts.

(D) less important in terms of impact than the compounds they produce.

22 In the eighth paragraph, what point does the writer make about the gut microbiota?

(A) It is a major factor in general health, independent of the presence of parasites.

(B) It tends to improve most noticeably when certain parasites are introduced.

(C) The consequences of deliberately introducing parasites to alter it are unpredictable.

(D) The research into its long-term response to parasites is still at an early stage.

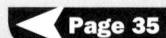
Genre and style

Your letter must be formal, with the technical level of language appropriate to the reader and with all the relevant case notes transformed accurately into full sentences.

1 Look at these case notes medical abbreviations. Write them as full sentences that might appear in the letter.

  1 Exercise: walking/cycling, 5x/week
  2 24 March 18: CBC & BMP
  3 Warfarin (Coumadin), 5 mg 1x/day, orally
  4 Headache – OTC paracetamol – ineffective

2 Read the extract from case notes below. Choose which sentence most accurately communicates the notes.

> **20 Aug 17**
>
> ↑ Pain, BP and breathing difficult; treatment = 2x/day steroids via sub-cutaneous IV

  1 On 20 August 17, the patient's pain had been increasing, and he had difficulty breathing. The treatment was two days of steroids via sub-cutaneous IV.
  2 On 20 August 17, the patient reported increasing pain, blood pressure and breathing difficulties. The treatment was steroids twice a day via sub-cutaneous IV.

Conciseness and clarity

1 Read the case notes. Decide where they belong in the timeline table. Today's date is 22 August 2021, and it is the date of discharge.

  a) Prescription: Warfarin (blood thinner/lowers blood pressure), ACE inhibitors (lowers blood pressure), beta-blockers (lowers blood pressure) & pain relief prn.
  b) Total hip replacement in 2000
  c) Angioplasty (insert stent); pt. recovered well
  d) Frequent bronchitis, smokers cough w phlegm; treatment = bronchodilators and steroids (inhaled)
  e) Acute myocardial infarction: tightness in chest; pain in chest, back, jaw (< 2mins); sweating; tachycardia (105 BPM).
  f) Increase healthy activity: walking 30 mins/day, swimming 1x/week, & no weightlifting
  g) Diagnosis from ECG; family informed
  h) Decrease smoking & alcohol; currently 3 standard drinks/day, and 1 pack of cigarettes/day

> **Tip!** Putting the case notes into a timeline can help you decide which events/details can be grouped together and summarised for inclusion in your letter.

> **Tip!** Your letter should only include information that is relevant to the case. Here the total hip replacement is not relevant to the reason for admission or discharge, and therefore should not be included.

Before admission (health background)	Upon admission (diagnosis)	During the stay (treatment)	Post discharge notes
(1)	(3)	(5)	(7) ....
(2)	(4)	(6)	(8) ....

2 Use the timeline to write the following information.

   1 A sentence or sentences that combine(s) admission details to explain the symptoms.

   2 A sentence or sentences that summarise(s) the treatment information related to lowering blood pressure.

   3 A sentence or sentences which summarise(s) what the patient should do post discharge.

> **Tip!** You can use the word count as a guide to help you decide if you are including too much or not enough information.

Language

1 Thinking about the patient above who has had an acute myocardial infarction, choose the best option(s) to complete the sentences. Sometimes both options might be correct.

   1 As his condition *has improved / was improving dramatically* in recent days, surgical intervention should only *be considering / be considered* if he has a relapse.

   2 The doctors *performed / were performing* an ECG which revealed that the patient *had suffered / had been suffering* a myocardial infarction.

   3 The patient *has recovered / has been recovered well* since a stent *inserted / was inserted* via angioplasty. To ensure the success of the surgery, warfarin, ACE inhibitors and beta-blockers *have prescribed / have been prescribed* to lower the patient's blood pressure.

   4 To maintain the progress that the patient has made, they *need / will need* to comply with the discharge plan. Specifically, weightlifting *must avoid / must be avoided*.

> **Tip!** Passives are common in formal letters as they de-personalise information and using them correctly in your letter may improve your language score.

2 Read the sentences below and chose the common error type each exemplifies. Then correct the errors. There may be more than one error in each sentence.

> spelling   word order   incorrect tense(s)   incorrect preposition   articles (*a/an*, *the*, or no article)
> too informal   punctuation   wrong word(s)

   1 Upon admission, Mr Spooner has been in a serious condition, but since then his health stabilised.

   2 Ms Grainger has suffered from the migraines since she was child.

   3 Renal function tests have been performed all were positive.

   4 The patient reacted adversely to the anastetic and was placed under observation.

   5 Advice by how the patient should reduce cholesterol has already been given by the doctor.

   6 An X-ray ruled out at the local clinic a Greenstick fracture.

   7 I am writting to refer Mr Green, a 26-year-old patient of mine, for farther examination of his temporomandibular joint.

   8 Mrs Ye presented at a clinic this morning, where she fainted.

> **Tip!** Under exam conditions, it is easy to make simple mistakes when you write that could affect your score. Always leave time at the end to check your letter.

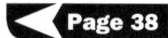 **Page 38** *Action plan*

TIME ALLOWED: **READING TIME: 5 MINUTES**
                   WRITING TIME: 40 MINUTES

Read the case notes and complete the writing task which follows.

Notes:

Assume that today's date is 10 March 2019.
Ms Sandra Green is a regular patient of yours at your general practice.

PATIENT DETAILS:

Name:	Ms Sandra Green
DOB:	08 February 2000 (19 y.o.)
Address:	132 Nutwood St, Newtown

Social background:	Saleswoman, IT company (= stressful job)
	Limited socialising (long work hours)
	Non-smoker & non-drinker
	Only child, lives alone
	Tennis practice/matches 2x/wk

Family History:	Father – recurring gout (managed w. diet plan)
	Mother – hypercholesteroliema (low cholesterol diet)

Medical history:	Nil significant, no surgeries
	2015: Anorexia Nervosa (A.N.), BMI =15.2
	Pt. taken by parents to outpatient clinic appts
	Pt. recovered w psychotherapy & nutritional support

> **Tip!** Look over all the dates given in the case notes. Try to create a timeline in your mind during reading time and eliminate any dates that are not relevant to the continuation of care.

> **Tip!** Rather than simply listing the important information in separate sentences, try to show how it is linked through complex sentences. For instance, using relative clauses like "which shows" to explain test results.

| Current medication: | Herbal supplements from naturopath: gingko biloba & ginseng (both to ↓stress) |
| | Over-the-counter laxatives |

Treatment record

20 Feb 2019:	Presenting complaint: constipation (last 2 wks)
	Subjective: fatigue, bloating, no menstrual irregularities
	Objective: no distention visible, BP = 80/60, weight = 55 kg, height = 173 cm, BMI = 18.4
	Discussion: pt. requests strong laxatives, OTC laxatives ineffective
	Wants to 'look her best', role is 'very image focused'
	Pt. admitted to counting calories to maintain weight (approx. 1700/day)
	Laxative request refused; suspected A.N. relapse
	Advice: ↑fibre in diet (e.g. oats, vegetables & legumes) & ↑calories (sport levels)
	CBC & BMP (Basic Medical Panel) ordered

20 March 2019:	Blood test results: low FE, calcium, potassium, T3 & T4 = ?low nutrient level in diet
	Subjective: tearfulness, depressed mood, ↓energy
	Repeated request for laxatives
	Objective: BP = 80/60, weight = 53 kg, BMI = 17.7
	Discussion:
	Explained possible complications re long-term laxative use = IBS, colon infection & liver damage
	Pt. admits: laxatives for weight loss & may be 'slipping into old habits' = Calorie intake = approx. 1500/day
	Pt. requests A.N. support

| **Plan:** | Refer to psychiatrist |
| | Multidisciplinary team (psychiatrist to organise): GP, psychiatrist & nutritionist |

Writing Task:

Using the information in the case notes, write a letter of referral to Dr Smith, Psychiatrist, summarising Ms Green's relevant medical history, outlining your concerns and requesting further management. Address the letter to Dr John Smith, Psychiatrist, Newtown Hospital, 123 High Street, Newtown.

In your answer:

- **Expand the relevant notes into complete sentences**
- **Do not use note form**
- **Use letter format**

The body of the letter should be approximately 180–200 words.

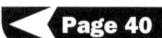 **Page 40**   *Task information*

Patient language

Patients in Part A often speak in everyday language to refer to symptoms, body parts and feelings. However, the information on the patient notes tends to be more formal medical language. You need to be able to match the meaning of what the patient says to the information on the notes as you listen, so you can follow the audio and anticipate when answers are coming.

> **Tip!** The answers for the gaps are always words / phrases you hear directly in the audio extract. You shouldn't change their form or make them into more medically correct language.

1 Look at the following sets of words and phrases which express the same idea. In each set, underline the one which is less likely to be used by the patient and more likely to appear in the patient notes.

1 pee / urine
2 vomiting / throwing up
3 getting better / improving
4 given / prescribed

5 acute (pain) / stabbing (pain)
6 deteriorated / got worse
7 insomnia / can't sleep / sleepless nights
8 useless / ineffective / a waste of time

2 Look at the words in the box which refer to quantity, frequency or duration and put them in the correct column.

| hardly ever | never-ending | insufficient | excessive |

Common language patient may use in audio	Formal (medical language) more likely in patient notes
	persistent / chronic
not enough	
too much	
	infrequently

3  Listen to the six short extracts of patients explaining how they feel. Choose an appropriate adjective from the box below to summarise how they are feeling. The first one has been done for you.

> **Tip!** Sometimes the patient will give an extended explanation of their feelings or situation, but this may be written in the patient notes as a single word.

| stressed | unwell | ~~nauseous~~ | frightened | fed up | confused |

1 ......*nauseous*........

2 ....

3 ....

4 ....

5 ....

6 ....

Giving full answers

Sometimes, in order to complete a gap and get the mark, you need to write the full name of a condition, treatment, body part, etc., because it contains important information/detail and the answer may be incomplete without it.

1 Look at the five sentences below and underline the full names of the conditions, body parts and treatments in each. The first one has been done for you as an example.

> **Tip!** Look at question 2 here. If you only write 'dermatitis' you are not being specific enough as there are many types (contact, atopic, seborrheic, etc.) and the audio will almost always state which type.

   1 So, I was diagnosed with <u>type 1 diabetes</u> at the age of five.
   2 She said it looked like contact dermatitis.
   3 I know my mum had an early menopause.
   4 I'm just using a topical corticosteroid twice a day.
   5 I was wondering – is there anything we can do about these stretch marks?

2  Now listen to five speakers and complete the notes with the full name of the condition, treatment or body part mentioned.

   1 .... (20 years)
   2 .... most painful.
   3 .... (18 months ago)
   4 recent .... (osteoporosis)
   5 barium swallow test excluded ....

> **Tip!** If the missing information is a limb or part of limb, e.g., knee, you need to say which knee it is to answer correctly.

3 Look at the extract from the patient notes below. For each gap, decide what kind of information (a–d) you think is missing that you need to listen for in the audio extract.

   a) medical conditions   **c)** parts of the body
   b) medicines or treatments   **d)** other

Tests
   • **(7)** .... (two weeks ago)
   • initial ESR test: elevated inflammation levels
   • **(8)** .... confirmed

Triggers
   • **(9)** .... (now mainly related to studies)
   • cold weather
   • **(10)** .... (increase in past 12 months)

Current medication
   • **(11)** .... (x2 daily)
   • antihistamine p.r.n.

Patient concerns
   • patches may be **(12)** ....
   • impact of chronic condition on life
   • impact on ability to manage anxiety
     if condition progresses

---

4   Now listen and complete the rest of the extract. Make sure you write the full names of conditions/treatments/medicines where required.

◄ Page 42 *Action plan*

Part A

In this part of the test, you'll hear two different extracts. In each extract, a health professional is talking to a patient.

  For **questions 1–24**, complete the notes with information that you hear.

Now, look at the notes for extract one.

Extract 1: Questions 1–12

You hear a dietician talking to a patient called Carina Bretby. For **questions 1–12**, complete the notes with a word or short phrase that you hear.

You now have thirty seconds to look at the notes.

Patient   Carina Bretby

Medical history   • surgery for **(1)** _____ (ten years ago)
                    • biopsy for suspected **(2)** _____
                      (eight years ago)

Onset of symptoms (gradual)
                    • generalised fatigue – later combined with sleeplessness
                      – exacerbated by **(3)** _____ and
                        frequent urination
                    • partial loss of taste – **(4)** _____ foods
                      affected
                    • began to feel **(5)** _____ - loss of grip
                      and co-ordination
                    • itchiness – mostly affected nose and skin around
                      (6) _____
                    • persistent ulcer on **(7)** _____

Diagnosis & treatment • iron deficiency suspected – follows a
                      (8) _____ diet
                    • **(9)** _____ ruled out – blood test
                      revealed pernicious anaemia
                    • daily B12 supplements initially – gradually reduced to eleven-
                      week intervals
                    • began to experience **(10)** _____ by
                      week nine
                    • some breathlessness by week ten

Current concerns   • temporary infertility resolved by B12 treatment
                    • pregnant – taking **(11)** _____
                      supplement in addition to folic acid
                    • concerned about risk of **(12)** _____ in
                      child (requests dietary advice)

Extract 2: Questions 13–24

You hear a doctor at a student health centre talking to a patient called Rory Aziz. For **questions 13–24**, complete the notes with a word or short phrase that you hear.

You now have thirty seconds to look at the notes.

Patient:	Rory Aziz (second-year student)

Onset of symptoms
- repeated episodes of **(13)** _____ during first weeks of school (aged 5)

- recalls frequent sensation of '**(14)** _____' in stomach as a child

- repeated bouts of anxiety in adolescence
    - characterised by what he calls '**(15)** _____' regarding future events
    - admits to finding anxious thoughts **(16)** _____ at that time

- some improvement in late teens

Symptoms at college
- experienced a **(17)** _____ at night
    - attributed to high intake of caffeine
    - symptoms included palpitations, tingling and sensation of **(18)** _____

- subsequently experienced daytime **(19)** _____ and light headedness
    - accompanied by dry mouth and excessive **(20)** _____

Diagnosis and treatment
- blood tests ruled out anaemia and **(21)** _____

- diagnosis of GAD (generalised anxiety disorder)

- CBT (four months) – effective in reducing symptoms

Current concerns
- would like to try **(22)** _____ therapy

- requests information about medication - mentions **(23)** _____
    - concerned about side effects

- has become aware of a **(24)** _____ (back of head)

Advice

13 What type of symptoms can be described as 'episodes' in children?

14 The missing word is part of a common expression related to anxiety.

15 The notes say 'in adolescence', but in the audio Rory says 'in my teens.' Listen for two words.

16 After he says 'Looking back', you hear a word that describes his anxious thoughts.

17 Read the whole bullet point as Rory talks about his coffee (caffeine) intake before you hear the answer.

18 The word you're listening for comes after he's talked about his heart and tingling in his body.

19 Listen for a noun connected to light headedness.

20 Rory says, 'I had other symptoms too', which matches 'accompanied by' in the notes.

21 Listen for a two-word condition a blood test might rule out.

22 Because Rory isn't sure that he's got the right term, he says 'What they call' before he says the answer.

23 Listen for a medication mentioned said to have 'a few side effects'.

24 What might Rory have noticed on the back of his head? Think of some possible symptoms.

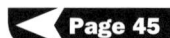 **Page 45** *Task information*

Listening for meaning

For each extract in Part B, you may hear something relating to the ideas in each of the answer options in the recording. However, you're listening for the answer to a specific question about what you hear. Make sure that the option you choose correctly answers the question you've been asked.

1  Look at the audio transcript below as you listen to the recording. Parts of the transcript that include ideas in the options have been underlined. Choose the correct option to answer the question. Can you explain why the other options are incorrect?

You hear a briefing for staff in a primary-care practice about a new online prescription service.

What is the main aim of the service?

A to enhance patients' understanding of their medication

B to improve the experience offered to certain patients

C to increase the number of patients who can be seen

> **Tip!** In a medical workplace, you don't just focus on the words that are said to you, but also on how they are said as the intonation and stress help you understand what someone is communicating. The same applies to Part B Listening.

> We're starting the new online prescription service today, and we're encouraging all our patients to sign up for it. **Option B:** Basically, we're giving them this leaflet that explains everything. We hope it will make things a lot easier for the most vulnerable, because they can have their prescriptions delivered, instead of having to go to the pharmacy and wait in the queue, something which can actually be really difficult for people who work too. **Option C:** There'll also be less need for personal contact, so we should have fewer people coming into the practice – which is an added bonus. **Option A:** But, obviously we still do have some people who really rely on explanations from the pharmacist and face-to-face contact, so rather than assuming that people know how to manage their prescription – what to expect and how to take it and so on – if you have any doubts, tell them to call in at the pharmacy to discuss things the first time they use the service.

2  Look at the audio transcript as you listen to the recording. Focus on the pronunciation. Underline any words that you think are emphasised. How do these emphasised words help you to know which is the correct option?

> Basically, we're giving them this leaflet that explains everything. We hope it will make things a lot easier for the most vulnerable, because they can have their prescriptions delivered, instead of having to go to the pharmacy and wait in the queue, something which can actually be really difficult for people who work too.

Recognising main versus supporting points

1  Read the information box and answer the question below it. Listen to a short extract and choose the line of dialogue that answers the question (the main idea of what is said).

> **The main idea/point/purpose/function in the recording may be**
> **i.** given using a different type of language from the option that matches it.
> **ii.** not directly stated, but may be a summary of what is being said.
> **iii.** supported by explanations, examples, descriptions, etc.
> **iv.** emphasised in some way by the speaker's intonation.
>
> **Supporting information may be**
> **i.** a single detail or aspect of the main point, such as an explanation of or reason for the main point or an example to clarify the main point.
> **ii.** incidental information which is not necessarily related the main point.

What is the nurse who's speaking emphasising about checking the wound?

a) *'It might be a good idea to do it right at the beginning of both shifts.'*

b) *'It definitely must be checked at least twice a day, mornings and evenings.'*

2  Read the question below and listen to the audio recording. Write down what you think the hospital nurse is doing. Think about the overall purpose of everything she says in terms of the patient and listen carefully to her pronunciation.

You hear a hospital nurse talking to a patient who's about to be discharged.
What is the nurse doing?

3 Now look at the answer options. Which one best matches what you wrote down.

    A giving the patient information about travel arrangements
    B explaining some documentation to the patient
    C outlining the patient's follow-up care

4 Now read the audio transcript and listen to the recording again. Sections that relate to each of the answer options has been underlined and labelled. For each section, think about whether the speaker is expressing the main idea (the correct answer) or supporting ideas.

> **Nurse:** Hello, Mr Daniels, good news – **(Option B)** <u>I'm just about to fill out all your paperwork for you and then you can be discharged.</u> The doctor needs to see you first, to make sure she's happy that the antibiotics are working and she's on her way round now. **(Option C)** <u>So, I just want to run through what's going to happen afterwards with the home-visiting team and make sure you're happy.</u>
> **Mr Daniels:** That would be great.
> **Nurse: (Option A)** <u>Now you've said that your daughter's coming to pick you up and drive you home, which is great.</u> So, this evening a care assistant will meet you at home and she or one of her colleagues will be popping round twice a day to see how you're getting on with your medications, check you're comfortable and have everything you need. She'll also communicate with your doctor if there are any concerns or anything you're worried about. How does that sound?
> **Mr Daniels:** Yes, that's all pretty clear.

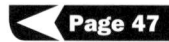

◀ Page 47 *Action plan*

Part B

In this part of the test, you'll hear six different extracts. In each extract, you'll hear people talking in a different healthcare setting.

For **questions 25–30**, choose the answer (**A, B** or **C**) which fits best according to what you hear. You'll have time to read each question before you listen. Complete your answers as you listen.

Now look at question 25.

Fill the circle in completely. Example:

---

25   You hear two hospital nurses handing over a patient at the change of shift.

What should the incoming nurse do first for the patient today?

(A)   organise some further investigations

(B)   implement agreed changes to his medication

(C)   begin to make arrangements for his discharge

26   You hear a senior care-home nurse briefing her team about patient mobility.

The video that they're going to watch will focus on

(A)   convincing patients of the need to move out of bed.

(B)   identifying which patients it is safe to move out of bed.

(C)   helping patients who would benefit from moving out of bed.

Advice

25 *One of the options has already taken place and another is for tomorrow. What planned activity does the incoming colleague need to action today?*

26 *The nurse uses the word 'video' at the start, but later talks about 'the clip I've selected'. Listen for what the clip focuses on and match that to one of the options.*

27 You hear a community nurse talking to a patient.

What is the patient most concerned about?

(A) the level of discomfort that he's experiencing

(B) how certain types of treatment might affect his work

(C) what the underlying causes of his symptoms might be

28 You hear a primary-care doctor talking to a practice nurse about a patient.

What is the doctor requesting?

(A) regular feedback on the patient's progress

(B) an informal assessment of the patient's mental state

(C) advice on whether home visits would be more appropriate

29 You hear a community pharmacist talking to a patient.

What concerns the patient about his medication?

(A) whether he's understood the dosage instructions

(B) whether he has sufficient supplies for his needs

(C) whether the correct type has been supplied

30 You hear part of a safety briefing on a hospital ward on the subject of hand hygiene.

What is the speaker doing?

(A) recommending a newly published training tool

(B) announcing a new way of accessing a standard training tool

(C) suggesting a training tool to address a new problem that's arisen

Advice

27 The expression 'The thing is' introduces the aspect of his finger problem that concerns him most.

28 Listen for the language the doctor uses to make a polite request using a modal verb.

29 Listen to the whole story the patient tells before deciding which option best matches what he's concerned about.

30 Note that all the options have the word 'new.' Listen for what is 'new' about the package the speaker is talking about.

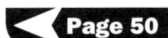 **Page 50**   *Task information*

Listening for meaning

Use the preparation time to think carefully about the meaning of each answer option. You're not listening for key words in the answer options, but for whether the ideas you hear match the overall meaning of an option AND answer the question.

1   Look at the context sentence and question 3 from the sample Part C listening extract we looked at in Training Test 1. Key words in the question stem and answer options have been underlined. Answer the questions 1–4.

You hear an interview with a nurse educator called Marika Alford, who's talking about a project to help student nurses develop the skills associated with delivering bad news.

3   Marika feels that <u>student nurses receive little training</u> in delivering bad news <u>because</u>
   A the <u>skills</u> tend to be <u>undervalued generally</u>.
   B it's <u>difficult</u> to <u>organise</u> any <u>meaningful practice</u>.
   C <u>patients</u> are <u>reluctant</u> for <u>consultations</u> to be <u>observed</u>.

   1   If something is 'undervalued generally', what does that tell us about how people feel about it?
   2   What reasons can you think of for why 'bad news' skills training might be difficult to organise?
   3   What is meant by 'meaningful practice' of skills?
   4   If someone is 'reluctant' about something, how do they feel about it?

2      Now listen to the section of the recording and read the audio transcript. The part of the recording that contains the answer is underlined. Think about your answers to Exercise 1 and decide which option best summarises the meaning of the reason Marika gives.

Interviewer: So why aren't nurses given training in this?
Marika: What we realised is that factors combine to prevent student nurses getting the opportunity to develop these skills. <u>Typically, in practice placements, students get to sit in on medical procedures and consultations as they take place, often with the patient's permission. But there's a general feeling that this would be neither practical nor fair on patients in this particular context. So, it's not so much that these skills are thought unimportant, but rather than they can only be developed in the actual situation. It's easy enough to see why in a busy course programme, the logistics rule this out.</u> But we wanted to find a way to develop these skills and encourage best practice.

Tip! The correct answer option may summarise the overall meaning of the corresponding section of the recording, rather than just a single sentence within it.

3  Now look at question 4. The correct answer is option C. Listen to the corresponding section of the audio recording and then read the transcript. Underline the part of the transcript that you think corresponds to option C.

4 Why did Marika's team decide to use simulations as part of the project?

    A These had worked well in other medical contexts.
    B The use of audio-visual material proved ineffective.
    C It gave participants insights into the patient experience.

> **Interviewer:** And I think you chose to use simulations – why was that?
> **Marika:** That's right. Clearly participation in actual face-to-face consultations was out of the question. Video was an option, but there's still the problem of actually gathering authentic material. Actors pretending to be patients can provide a suitable model for students to watch, but that's not the same as getting actual practice. Simulations seemed to be the answer, with nurses in pairs alternately playing the role of either the health professional or the patient. What convinced us was that this method also gives the student nurses a chance to see how the situation feels from different perspectives. Simulation is widely used in medicine, but usually for critical clinical events – like cardiac arrests or traumatic injuries – and not generally for communication skills – so this was something of a new departure.

4  Now look at question 5. Listen to the corresponding section of the audio recording. The parts of the transcript that contain ideas expressed in the options are underlined. First, decide which answer option is correct. Then look at the incorrect options. Can you explain why they are incorrect?

> **Tip!** You may hear words or ideas that correspond to incorrect answer options. Listen carefully to decide if the idea expressed in an option is the same as the idea expressed by the speaker AND answers the question.

5 What aspect of the training did Marika find surprisingly successful?

    A hearing about participants' own experiences
    B participants providing some of the input material
    C using a learning tool designed for another purpose

> **Interviewer:** But it was actually very successful.
> **Marika:** That's right. We set up a three-stage interactive workshop.
> **Option A:** Firstly, students were asked to relate any experiences they'd had of breaking bad news – and this did turn out to be fairly limited. **Option C:** Next, we moved onto theory, using a well-established teaching tool – the ABCDE mnemonic – each letter stands for one step in the process of breaking bad news. It's a sound approach and it proved to be a good choice.
> **Option B:** Then the students came up with scenarios of their own and took it in turns to act these out in each of the roles. We weren't sure how this phase would go, but actually it exceeded all expectations. When students reported back to the group, there was a lot of useful discussion.

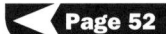

Test 2 Exam practice   Listening   Part C

Page 52 *Action plan*

Part C

In this part of the test, you'll hear two different extracts. In each extract, you'll hear health professionals talking about aspects of their work.

For **questions 31–42**, choose the answer (**A, B** or **C**) which fits best according to what you hear. Complete your answers as you listen.

Now look at extract one.

Fill the circle in completely. Example:

Extract 1: Questions 31–36

You hear a nurse called Maya Leyden giving a presentation on the subject of hospital visiting times.

You now have 90 seconds to read **questions 31–36**.

31   What point does Maya make about historical reasons for restricting hospital visiting times?

   (A)   They've all been discounted by research.

   (B)   Some aspects of them are still justifiable.

   (C)   More needs to be done to establish their validity.

32   Maya points to evidence that the policy of protecting rest and mealtimes

   (A)   was largely introduced for the wrong reasons.

   (B)   still has a place in some healthcare settings.

   (C)   hasn't been shown to be beneficial.

> **Advice**
>
> **31** *After introducing her topic, Maya takes a breath and begins with the word 'historically'. This matches the 'historical reasons' that this question asks about.*
>
> **32** *The key idea here is evidence. Listen for what Maya says about 'a recent systematic review'.*

33 Maya suggests that staff concerns about open visiting

- (A) need to be addressed through training.
- (B) should inform a review of certain procedures.
- (C) have to be investigated as valid reasons for restricting it.

34 Maya feels that involving family members directly in patient care

- (A) can provide useful insights for health professionals.
- (B) is more appropriate in some settings than others.
- (C) needs to be handled on a case-by-case basis.

35 How does Maya respond to fears that open visiting might be a 'free for all'?

- (A) She questions whether these are reasonable concerns.
- (B) She quotes research that shows this not to be the case.
- (C) She suggests how potential issues might be addressed.

36 In her conclusion, Maya suggests that decisions on hospital visiting times should

- (A) be an issue for public consultation.
- (B) have their basis in sound research findings.
- (C) try to accommodate the views of all concerned.

Advice

33 You're listening for what Maya 'suggests'. Listen for when she says: 'This is an issue, but maybe …' after which you hear her point of view.

34 Listen for what Maya says about the findings of a recent study. Her view is confirmed by what she says about paediatrics and informal care situations.

35 Focus on the studies she talks about and what she says afterwards.

36 Maya signals that she's coming to the end of her presentation with words 'So what conclusions can we come to?' Listen to everything she says after this.

Extract 2: Questions 37–42

You hear an interview with a tissue viability nurse called Matteo Moran who is talking about the use of maggot therapy in debridement.

You now have 90 seconds to read **questions 37–42**.

37 What surprises Matteo about the early development of maggot therapy?

    Ⓐ how long it has actually been in use

    Ⓑ the way its potential was first recognised

    Ⓒ why its initial success was relatively short-lived

38 For Matteo, the main advantage of maggot therapy over other methods of debridement is that

    Ⓐ radical surgery is more often avoided.

    Ⓑ there are marked savings in both time and money.

    Ⓒ there is a reduced need for certain types of medication.

39 Matteo explains that maggot therapy isn't currently more widely used due to

    Ⓐ a lack of specialist staff to administer it.

    Ⓑ concerns about possible complications.

    Ⓒ the need to ensure reliable supplies.

40 How do most of Matteo's patients feel about receiving maggot therapy?

    Ⓐ enthusiastic at the prospect of recovery

    Ⓑ concerned about what people may think

    Ⓒ resigned to putting up with the indignity

Advice

37 You're listening for what surprises Matteo. He uses the word 'incredible' to introduce this idea.

38 All three are mentioned as advantages, but he says 'crucially from my point of view' to introduce what he sees as the main advantage.

39 This question is asking you for a reason. Matteo talks about all three options, but which of these does he say is 'a barrier to more widespread use.'

40 The question is asking you about Matteo's patients in particular – not patients in general. Listen for his patients' attitude once the treatment is underway and the reason that follows.

41 Research into the attitude of UK healthcare staff towards the therapy suggests that

- (A) the majority are unwilling to administer it.

- (B) some might need extra support to overcome their initial objections.

- (C) opposition to it may be slowing its adoption.

42 How does Matteo view the future of maggot therapy?

- (A) The arguments in its favour are gaining ground.

- (B) It's most likely to be used alongside existing methods.

- (C) Further research is needed to finally establish its worth.

Advice

41 *Be careful. Two of the options relate to a hypothetical point that is made and are as such are incorrect. Which option relates to a conclusion drawn based on the UK research?*

42 *Ideas in all three options are mentioned, but which summarises Mateo's view?*

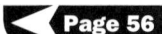 **Page 56** *Task information*

Therapeutic communication skills

Use therapeutic communication during the role plays to show your patient-focused manner as you will be assessed on how well you do this.

1  You are going to hear a dialogue between a doctor and a patient divided into three sections. In each section, the doctor uses one or more of the following therapeutic communication skills. Listen and tick (✓) the therapeutic communication skill(s) demonstrated. The first one has been done as an example.

Therapeutic communication skill	Section 1	Section 2	Section 3
Showing empathy for the patient's feelings/situation e.g., *That must be very difficult.*	✓		
Using a non-judgmental approach e.g., *It can be hard to lose weight, but many people find…*			
Showing a respectful attitude e.g., *You can decide which option works best for you.*	✓		
Exploring the patient's ideas/concerns/expectations e.g., *Can you tell me a little more about that?*	✓		
Relating explanations to patient's own feelings/experience e.g., *You mentioned earlier that you own a dog. Perhaps you could try taking him for walks each day to boost your physical activity.*			

2 Listen again and note down any phrases the doctor uses demonstrating the skills you identified. Read the audio transcript if necessary.

Giving advice vs giving instructions

When the role play asks you to give instructions, you can be quite direct with the patient/carer, e.g., *Take these tablets twice daily.* When you give advice, use more polite or indirect language. *Advice tasks will start with verbs such as Advise, Recommend,* and *Emphasise importance of.*

1  Listen to a doctor giving advice to patients and write the missing phrases that introduce the advice.

1 .... reduce your caffeine intake as coffee can make your heartburn worse.

2 .... do only light exercises until the stitches are removed.

3 .... wash your hands before using the glucometer because otherwise the result could be inaccurate.

4 .... book a follow-up appointment in two weeks?

5 .... reduce your alcohol intake as this aggravates your condition.

6 .... keep a diary of when the symptoms flare up.

> **Tip!** Tasks which begin with 'Emphasise importance of…' or 'Stress the need for…' will require stronger language than 'Advise' or 'Recommend'.

2   Look at the phrases you wrote in Exercise 1. Which ones would you use when the advice/recommendations need to be stronger?

3   Look at the advice tasks in the role card extract below. Make notes on how you will advise the patient.
- Advise patient on dietary modifications (e.g., decreased salt/saturated fat intake, increased fresh fruit/vegetables, etc.).
- Emphasise importance of physical activity (e.g., weight management, improved mood/energy, better sleep, etc.).

4    Listen to a doctor completing the tasks on the role card. Compare the doctor's recommendations with your own notes. Read the audio transcript if necessary. Can you find any examples of when the doctor uses phrases from Exercise 1?

Resolving the point of tension

In every role play, there is a conflict of some kind, which you need to resolve. Again, a patient-focused approach is required to deal with this.

1   Read each point of tension below. Cross (✗) the approach that you think would be least effective in resolving the point of tension.
   1   The patient is reluctant to follow your advice.
      a)   Tell the patient directly that he/she has no choice.
      b)   Show empathy to the patient's situation or concerns.
      c)   Emphasise the benefits of the proposed advice.
   2   The patient has been non-compliant in taking his/her medication.
      a)   Highlight the risks of medication non-compliance.
      b)   Offer suggestions on ways of improving compliance.
      c)   Accuse the patient of having poor self-discipline and putting their health at risk.

> **Tip!** Sometimes a combination of approaches may be helpful in resolving the point of tension.

2    Listen to a doctor resolving the points of tension in Exercise 1 and circle the phrase used for each.

   1   **a)**   *I can appreciate that it's not easy to..., but...*
      b)   *I understand how difficult it can be to..., but...*
   2   **a)**   *Please make sure that you...*
      b)   *It's really important to...*

3    Listen again to the points of tension from Exercise 2. Pause the audio after each patient has spoken. Practise resolving each point of tension using the relevant approaches and/or phrases from Exercises 1 and 2.

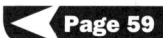 **Page 59** *Action plan*

Note that you are also provided with the interlocutor's role card here. In the actual exam, you will only see your role card.

OET SAMPLE TEST

ROLEPLAYER CARD NO. 1	MEDICINE

SETTING   Doctor's Clinic

PATIENT   You are 48 years old and have very sore feet. The doctor has just finished examining your feet.

TASK
- When asked, say your feet started hurting about four months ago. It feels like a burning pain. The pain is most intense in the heels. The pain is there all the time, but it's worse when you first get out of bed.
- When asked, say you work as a chef and you have to stand up all day. You don't have time for any exercise outside of work. You often skip meals during the day, and you often eat fast food on your drive home from work. You don't have any other health conditions or take medications.
- Say you'll follow the self-care advice. Ask how long it will take to feel better.
- Say that you've tried to lose weight before but had no success, so there's no point trying again.
- Say that you'll try again to lose some weight. You'll look for a weight loss support group in your area.

© Cambridge Boxhill Language Assessment (2022)   SAMPLE TEST

OET SAMPLE TEST

CANDIDATE CARD NO. 1	MEDICINE

SETTING   Doctor's Clinic

DOCTOR   This 48-year-old obese patient is seeing you today to talk about foot pain. You have just finished examining the patient's feet. You diagnose plantar fasciitis.

TASK
- Find out more details about patient's foot pain (e.g., onset, pain characteristics, constant/ intermittent, etc.).
- Explore patient's lifestyle (e.g., work, exercise, diet, health conditions, medications, etc.).
- Give diagnosis of plantar fasciitis (e.g., ligament inflammation, caused by excess pressure on feet, etc.). Advise on self-care (e.g., stretching, supportive shoes, rest, ice, ibuprofen, etc.).
- Give likely timescale for recovery (e.g., up to 6 months, dependent on self-care compliance, etc.). Stress importance of weight loss (e.g., pressure/inflammation reduction in feet, overall health benefit, etc.).
- Warn of risks of maintaining current weight (e.g., more/ongoing foot problems, further/more serious health issues, etc.). Make recommendations for weight loss (e.g., support groups/ programmes, dietary sheets, etc.).

© Cambridge Boxhill Language Assessment (2022)   SAMPLE TEST

ROLEPLAYER CARD NO. 2   **MEDICINE**

SETTING	Emergency Department
CARER	You have brought your four-year-old daughter to the hospital because she's been vomiting and feverish for ten hours. Your daughter has been triaged by the nurse, and her urine has been collected for testing. The doctor sees you to talk about your daughter's condition. Your daughter is not present during this discussion.
TASK	• When asked, say your daughter had a slight stomach ache last night but no diarrhoea. • When asked, say your daughter recently started using the toilet independently, so you haven't been paying attention to her toileting habits. • Say you're glad she's being treated, but you don't think the diagnosis is correct. You really think it's gastroenteritis because your daughter's friend had it. • Say you accept your daughter has a urinary tract infection. Ask how long she will have to stay in hospital. • Say you will call a family member to bring an overnight bag so that you can stay with her.

© Cambridge Boxhill Language Assessment (2022)   SAMPLE TEST

OET SAMPLE TEST

CANDIDATE CARD NO. 2   **MEDICINE**

SETTING	Emergency Department
DOCTOR	This parent has brought in his/her four-year-old daughter with a ten-hour history of vomiting and fever. The child was triaged by the nurse and a urine culture was taken. Preliminary urinalysis indicates the presence of leukocytes. You have read the notes and are now going to talk to the parent. The child is not present during this discussion.
TASK	• Find out about any other symptoms in child (e.g., stomach cramps, diarrhoea, etc.). • Explore child's recent toileting history (e.g., frequency, urgency, dysuria, etc.). • Give preliminary diagnosis of urinary tract infection (e.g., rectal bacteria entering urinary tract, some children susceptible, associated vomiting/fever, etc.). Outline management (e.g., immediate paediatric ward admission, IV antibiotics for 48 hours, oral hydration fluids, etc.). • Justify diagnosis of urinary tract infection (e.g., suggestive presence of urine leukocytes, positive urine culture will confirm, no diarrhoea, risk factor – recently toilet trained, etc.). Find out about any further questions/concerns. • Give likely timescale for hospital admission (e.g., two days minimum, possibility of longer stay, etc). Explain next steps (e.g., child transfer to ward, begin treatment, etc.). Advise parent to stay with child.

© Cambridge Boxhill Language Assessment (2022)   SAMPLE TEST

Varicose Veins: Texts

Text A

Causes, risk factors and symptoms

Varicose veins are a chronic venous disease (CVD), which occurs when one-way valves in superficial, deep and/or perforating veins fail to close properly, causing blood to return and accumulate, rather than follow its normal path. This leads to a rise in venous pressure and distension, often resulting in veins being noticeable and presenting as twisted and enlarged.

Valvular dysfunction may be caused by congenital defects or weakening of the vein walls. Most commonly found in females and in the legs, common risk factors are advancing age, high body mass index, smoking, family history, history of trauma to lower extremities, previous venus thrombosis and pregnancy. It is estimated that 3 to 6 percent of people who have varicose veins in their lifetime will develop venous ulcers.

Some patients are asymptomatic, but others are impacted by painful, heavy, burning or throbbing legs, muscle cramps, and dry, itchy and thin skin over the affected area. Varicose veins often become more severe over time and can lead to complications such as alterations in skin pigmentation, bleeding, venous ulceration and tissue alteration and loss.

Text B

Initial examination

Take the patient's history:

Take a full history, bearing in mind that pelvic masses, trauma, and previous deep venous thrombosis are recognised causes. Determine whether the patient has aching leg pain (legs fatigue easily, feel heavy or are swollen). If they do, find out whether symptoms worsen as the day progresses especially with long periods of standing. In extreme cases, patients may describe venous claudication; acute, bursting pain on walking that can be alleviated by elevating the lower limbs. Patients with severe venous hypertension may complain of skin changes including venous eczema and ulceration, typically below the knee and above the ankle. Ask about any previous treatments.

Inspection:

Where possible, start with the patient standing with both legs bare to the groin. Gently press the affected areas, release, and observe the varicosities refill. Consider whether they are warmer than surrounding skin by using the back of the hand. Determine whether varicosities follow the long or short saphenous vein. Varicosities in the short saphenous vein are seen only below the knee and are usually at the back and to the outer edge of the leg (posterolateral). Long saphenous varicosities may be found along the length of the leg, usually on the medial aspect. Some people have a large accessory vein on the back (posterior) part of the thigh, which may become varicose.

Look for:

- Venous stars (venulectasias) - bluish vessels that may distend above skin surface. Usually 1–2 mm in diameter
- Superficial thrombophlebitis – red, painful lump
- Brown pigmentation caused by haemosiderin deposits
- Venous eczema – red or brown on lighter skin, dark brown, purple or grey on darkly pigmented skin*
- Ulceration and scarring from previous ulceration, especially in the gaiter area
- Lipodermatosclerosis; caused by chronic venous hypertension, results in sclerosis of skin and subcutaneous fat
- Scars from previous vein surgery (look for harvesting of vein grafts for coronary artery bypass grafting).

* venous eczema on darkly pigmented skin may be more difficult to see

Antibiotic treatment for Infected venous leg ulcers

Consider referring if the patient has a high risk of complications, infection of the lymph vessels, if infection is spreading and not responding to oral antibiotics or if the patient is unable to take oral antibiotics (where appropriate, explore locally available options for giving intravenous antibiotics at home or in a health centre, rather than in the hospital). Arrange urgent hospital referral if the patient has any symptoms or signs suggesting a more severe condition such as sepsis, necrotising fasciitis or osteomyelitis.

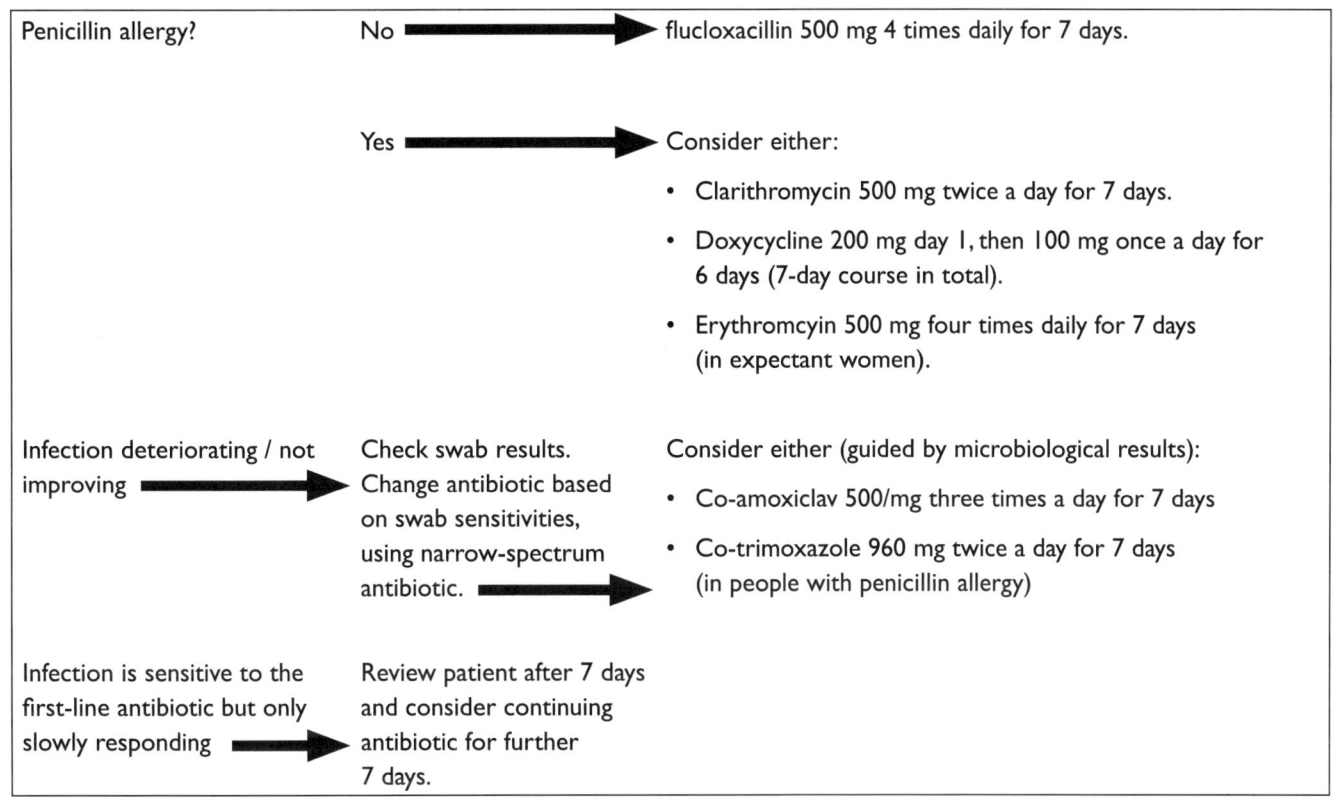

Penicillin allergy? No ⟶ flucloxacillin 500 mg 4 times daily for 7 days.

Yes ⟶ Consider either:

- Clarithromycin 500 mg twice a day for 7 days.
- Doxycycline 200 mg day 1, then 100 mg once a day for 6 days (7-day course in total).
- Erythromcyin 500 mg four times daily for 7 days (in expectant women).

Infection deteriorating / not improving ⟶ Check swab results. Change antibiotic based on swab sensitivities, using narrow-spectrum antibiotic. ⟶ Consider either (guided by microbiological results):

- Co-amoxiclav 500/mg three times a day for 7 days
- Co-trimoxazole 960 mg twice a day for 7 days (in people with penicillin allergy)

Infection is sensitive to the first-line antibiotic but only slowly responding ⟶ Review patient after 7 days and consider continuing antibiotic for further 7 days.

NB: routine long-term use of topical antiseptics and/or antimicrobials is not recommended

Text D

Interventional treatment options

Both **Endothermal ablation and Endovenous laser ablation** are minimally invasive catheter-based procedures in which thermal energy is delivered into the vein wall (intima), causing inflammation, which results in closure of the vein.

Endothermal ablation: The long saphenous vein is accessed above or below the knee, either percutaneously via an intravenous cannula/venepuncture sheath or via a small incision. The catheter is manually withdrawn at 2.5–3 cm/minute, and the vein wall temperature is maintained at 85°C.

Endovenous laser ablation:
A laser fibre is passed through the vein and positioned below the saphenofemoral junction. An anaesthetic agent is then injected and the fibre is slowly withdrawn while energy from a diode laser 810 or 940 NM wavelength is applied in short pulses. This is repeated along the full length of the vein until the long saphenous vein is sealed from the saphenofemoral junction to the point of access.

Ultrasound-guided foam sclerotherapy: Sclerosant foam is injected into the affected veins, causing an inflammatory reaction in the vein wall, scarring and eventual closure of the treated varicose vein. May be carried out under local anaesthesia. Compression bandages are applied after the procedure and are typically worn for between one and four weeks.

Duplex ultrasound guidance is the gold standard for assessment and diagnosis of superficial venous incompetence and is used to guide all the above interventions.

Part A

- Look at the four texts, **A–D**, in the separate **Text Booklet** that precedes the questions.

- For each question, **1–20**, look through the texts, **A–D**, to find the relevant information.

- Write your answers on the spaces provided in this **Question Paper**.

- Answer all the questions within the 15-minute time limit.

- Your answers should **only** be taken from texts **A–D** and must be correctly spelt.

Varicose Veins: Questions

Questions 1–7

For each question, **1–7**, decide which text (**A**, **B**, **C** or **D**) the information comes from. You may use any letter more than once.

In which text can you find information about

1	the best way to position a patient for an assessment?	_____
2	the best technology for visualising the veins?	_____
3	reasons why varicose veins protrude?	_____
4	why varicose veins can cause skin to change colour?	_____
5	when a patient requires specialist medical advice?	_____
6	how varicose veins are likely to progress?	_____
7	methods of blocking varicose veins?	_____

Questions 8–13

Answer each of the questions, **8–13**, with a word or short phrase from one of the texts. Each answer may include words, numbers or both.

8   How many flucloxacillin 500mg doses should be prescribed per day?

_____

9   Which immune system response is triggered by heating the wall of the vein?

_____

10   Which drug is a suitable alternative to Clarithromycin for patients who are pregnant?

_____

11   Which part of the body should you check for ulcer scars?

_____

12   What is drawn through the vein during endovenous laser ablation?

_____

13   Which procedure works by closing the long saphenous vein?

_____

Questions 14–20

Complete each of the sentences, **14–20**, with a word or short phrase from one of the texts. Each answer may include words, numbers or both.

14   When valves do not work efficiently, blood may reverse and
_____ instead of moving around the body.

15   Very high venous pressure can cause alterations to the _____,
usually on the lower leg.

16   If possible, IV treatment should be given in the patient's home or in a

_____

17   The dose of Doxycycline should be decreased to _____ a day
from day 2.

18   Venous claudication can be relieved by _____ the legs.

19   Venous eczema can be harder to spot in _____ skin.

20   Co-amoxiclav 500 mg should be taken _____ times daily.

Part B

In this part of the test, there are six short extracts relating to the work of health professionals.
For **questions 1–6**, choose the answer (**A**, **B** or **C**) which you think fits best according to the text.

Fill the circle in completely. Example:　Ⓐ Ⓑ Ⓒ

---

1 The purpose of this guideline on enteral feeding is to outline

　Ⓐ　the type of situations in which it might need to be used.

　Ⓑ　problems that can be encountered when implementing it.

　Ⓒ　the most appropriate way to assess a patient's suitability for it.

Guidelines: Enteral Feeding

Enteral feeding is the delivery of nutrients via a tube directly into the digestive tract. It is only necessary and/or desirable when nutritional needs cannot be met orally, for example, if a patient has an illness or injury, such as neck or head trauma, which prevents them from eating or swallowing food. Other indications include severe or sudden weight loss, poor absorptive capacity and/or high nutritional losses.

Patients with certain mental disorders (eg. anorexia nervosa, severe depression) may need to be fed enterally, if they lack the capacity to make informed decisions related to food or fluid intake. However, feeding against the patient's will should be an intervention of the last resort in the care and management of those with severe mental illnesses.

---

2 The guidelines on taking dogs to care settings state that in order to minimise the risk of infection

　Ⓐ　animals should be carefully examined beforehand.

　Ⓑ　patients should wear dressings on any open wounds.

　Ⓒ　no physical contact with the patient should be allowed.

Guidelines for infection prevention control – dogs visiting health and care settings

If the owner/handler or dog are unwell with diarrhoea and vomiting, or have been within the last 48 hours, they should not visit. This also applies to respiratory symptoms such as coughs and colds. Patients may only receive visits if any exposed surgical cuts or incisions have been covered. Both the dog and its owner must be up to date with all routine vaccinations. If the owner or dog develops a skin condition, prior advice should be sought from the local infection prevention and control team as to whether the visit should take place.

Although stroking and petting are permitted, the dog should not lick anyone or sit fully on the bed, particularly not near a person's face. If the dog is putting their feet on a bed, then an incontinence pad or similar should be put under their paws and discarded after each individual visit to avoid contamination

3 What is this memo saying about carbon monoxide monitoring for pregnant women?

(A) It is a valuable tool despite its limitations.

(B) Clinicians should decide for themselves whether to use it.

(C) The results should not be recorded if there are any doubts about their accuracy.

Memo: Using a carbon monoxide (CO) test to establish smoking status in pregnant women

Some women find it difficult to admit that they smoke because of social pressure not to. A carbon monoxide (CO) test is an immediate and non-invasive biochemical method for helping to ascertain whether they do or not. However, the best cut-off point for determining smoking status is unclear; some suggest a level as low as 3 parts per million (ppm), others use 6–10 ppm, as reliability can depend on circumstance. CO quickly disappears from expired breath (up to 50% in less than 4 hours) and conversely, external influences such as traffic emissions may lead to an elevated reading. As a result, low levels of smoking may go undetected and be indistinguishable from passive smoking. It is therefore advisable to use a low cut-off point to avoid missing someone who may need support.

---

4 The guidelines state that radiofrequency ablation of the soft palate for snoring

(A) could present risks for certain patients.

(B) might not be successful after one attempt.

(C) may lead to other types of sleep disturbance.

Radiofrequency ablation of the soft palate for snoring: guidelines for clinicians

The intention of radiofrequency ablation is to reduce airflow obstruction and vibration in the airway by scarring and tightening the soft palate. The procedure should only be used for patients whose snoring has been shown to be caused by abnormal movement of the soft palate and in whom sleep apnoea has been excluded. It is typically carried out under local anaesthesia in the outpatient department and may be combined with other procedures, such as uvulectomy or tonsillectomy. During the consent process, patients should be made aware of the potential need for further, multiple procedures at intervals of several weeks, if symptoms recur.

5 According to the memo, the new endometriosis service has been set up

   (A)   against a background of increasing referrals.

   (B)   as a direct result of patient pressure.

   (C)   in response to earlier failings.

Memo for family doctors

New endometriosis specialist service centre

Endometriosis is a complex and often misdiagnosed illness. Evidence suggests that care may at times have been delayed due to a lack of knowledge and understanding of the disease amongst health care workers. To address this situation, the hospital has set up a dedicated specialist centre which gives patients access to a multidisciplinary team, including a named colorectal surgeon and nurse specialist.

Initially, women will be seen by the specialist nurse and a full review of symptoms will be undertaken. The nurse will carry out any other incomplete or additional investigations and organise or perform a pelvic and renal ultrasound, if these are not supplied with the referral. Detailed literature will be provided and likely next steps discussed. If a laparoscopy is required, this will be organised directly by the nurse who will discuss each case with the doctor and multidisciplinary team.

---

6 The main aim of the guideline about delirium is to

   (A)   offer advice on how to recognise different types.

   (B)   stress the importance of monitoring symptoms.

   (C)   suggest ways of managing patients' behaviour.

Guideline for care home managers: identifying delirium

Delirium is a common clinical syndrome characterised by disturbed consciousness, cognitive function or perception, which has an acute onset and fluctuating course. It is a serious condition, associated with poor outcomes which can be prevented and treated if dealt with urgently. The majority of people living in care homes fall into the 'at risk' category.

Delirium can be hypoactive or hyperactive but some people show signs of both. People with hyperactive delirium have heightened arousal and can be restless, agitated and aggressive and those with hypoactive delirium become withdrawn, quiet and sleepy. It can be difficult to distinguish between delirium and dementia and some people may have both conditions. If clinical uncertainty exists over the diagnosis, the person should be treated initially for delirium.

In this part of the test, there are two texts about different aspects of healthcare. For **questions 27–42**, choose the answer (**A**, **B**, **C** or **D**) which you think fits best according to the text.

Fill the circle in completely. Example:

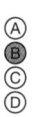

Text 1: Fibromyalgia

Affecting at least 1 in 40 people worldwide, fibromyalgia is a chronic illness characterised by widespread pain, muscle tenderness, and crippling fatigue. The cause of fibromyalgia is unknown, but many researchers believe that sufferers have a genetic predisposition to the illness, which is activated by a trigger such as stress, trauma or infection. Fibromyalgia has some features in common with autoimmune conditions such as rheumatoid arthritis and lupus, yet it does not qualify as an autoimmune disorder because scientists have so far been unable to identify the hallmark indicators: self-reactive T cells, autoantibodies and inflammation.

This standpoint looks set to change, however, in light of a new study published in the Journal of Clinical Investigation. The study, led by Dr David Andersson from the Institute of Psychiatry, Psychology and Neuroscience at King's College London, has found that fibromyalgia may be initiated by an autoimmune response that increases the activity of pain-sensing nerves throughout the body. These radical findings could potentially pave the way for more effective treatments for the millions of people affected.

Andersson and his colleagues harvested blood from 44 people with fibromyalgia and injected purified antibodies from them into mice. The mice rapidly became more sensitive to pressure and cold, and displayed reduced grip strength in their paws. Animals injected with antibodies from healthy people were unaffected. The mice recovered once the antibodies had been cleared from their systems, which took 2–3 weeks. This suggests that therapies such as plasma-exchange, which are designed to reduce antibody levels and which are available for other autoimmune disorders such as myasthenia gravis, may be effective in fibromyalgia patients.

This study opens up a line of research that so far has yielded few substantial results. 'Establishing that fibromyalgia is an autoimmune disorder will transform how we view the condition,' Dr Andersson said. 'Our work should give real hope to fibromyalgia patients. Current treatment tends to focus on gentle aerobic exercise, as well as drug and psychological therapies designed to manage pain. However, these have proven ineffective in most patients and have left behind an enormous unmet clinical need.'

The researchers have pointed out which aspects of the study warrant further investigation. 'The next step will be to identify what factors the symptom-inducing antibodies bind to,' says Prof Camilla Svensson from the Karolinska Institute in Sweden, who was also involved in the study. '**This** will then help us not only in terms of developing novel treatment strategies for fibromyalgia, but also of blood-based tests for diagnosis, which are missing today.'

Currently, there is no widely accepted medical test to diagnose fibromyalgia, so the prospect of a diagnostic biomarker is exciting. In 2010, the American College of Rheumatology (ACR) did publish a set of diagnostic criteria for fibromyalgia; however, its usefulness is questionable. A study in the journal Arthritis Care & Research found that doctors at a university rheumatology clinic over-diagnosed fibromyalgia in 43 patients out of 121 who met the criteria, and missed it entirely in 60 patients. In a large North American survey, 46% of fibromyalgia patients consulted 3–6 health care providers regarding their symptoms, before receiving a fibromyalgia diagnosis.

'Fibromyalgia can be underdiagnosed because we have to look for everything else first. On the other hand, fibromyalgia can also be over-diagnosed, because there's no specific blood work or imaging tests that we can do to diagnose it,' explains Dr Michelle Kahlenberg, associate professor in the division of rheumatology at the University of Michigan. Further confusion occurs because patients with fibromyalgia can also present with similar comorbidities such as rheumatoid arthritis or axial spondyloarthritis. These can be **red herrings**, leading doctors to assume that a patient's symptoms are caused by their existing disease, without recognizing that the patient's symptoms also put them in the category of fibromyalgia.

Fibromyalgia sufferers are understandably hopeful that Andersson and his colleagues' findings might shed some new light on this condition. Researchers and medical experts, on the other hand, are reserving their judgment. Dr Bronwyn Lennox Thompson, Senior Lecturer at the University of Otago, is mindful that the study was conducted on mice, which can be regarded as a shortcoming. 'Mice can't describe their experiences so we're inferring from their behavioural responses to short-term stimulation to humans who may be experiencing fibromyalgia for many years.' Des Quinn, the chair of Fibromyalgia Action UK, provided the following response to the study: 'The prospect of fibromyalgia being an autoimmune condition has been debated many times and this will add to that discussion. If these results can be replicated and expanded upon, then that would be extraordinary. However, the results need further confirmation and investigation before the outcomes can be applied universally.'

Text 1: Questions 7–14

7 What fact about fibromyalgia is the writer emphasising in the first paragraph?

(A) how difficult it is to know how many people have it

(B) how hard it is to distinguish it from other diseases

(C) how badly people's lives are affected by it

(D) how poorly understood it is

8 The study published in the Journal of Clinical Investigation

(A) caused controversy in the medical community.

(B) took far longer to complete than had been expected.

(C) provided support for an existing idea that has been difficult to prove.

(D) focused on treatment over diagnosis.

9   What does the writer tell us about Andersson's study in the third paragraph?

   (A)   The participants selected to take part in it were severely ill.

   (B)   The methodology presented a number of challenges to the team.

   (C)   The researchers were surprised by the strength of their findings.

   (D)   The results indicate a way forward in the treatment of fibromyalgia.

10   In the fourth paragraph, what point is made by Dr Andersson?

   (A)   Many attempts have been made to prove that fibromyalgia has an autoimmune basis.

   (B)   Previous investigation into fibromyalgia has only focused on pain management.

   (C)   Current fibromyalgia treatments are unsuccessful for many patients.

   (D)   Fibromyalgia sufferers are unable to tolerate prolonged physical exercise.

11   The word '**this**' in the fifth paragraph refers to

   (A)   the recognition of specific symptoms.

   (B)   the completion of the next step in the process.

   (C)   the development of a diagnostic test.

   (D)   the investigation into new treatments.

12   In the sixth paragraph, what do we learn about the ACR diagnostic criteria?

   (A)   Many doctors have complained about how unsatisfactory it is.

   (B)   Its usefulness depends on the experience of the doctor using it.

   (C)   There are doubts about the accuracy of clinical research into its use.

   (D)   It is limited in its effectiveness to diagnose fibromyalgia.

13 The writer refers to '**red herrings**' to highlight the way

- Ⓐ doctors can be misled by what patients say.

- Ⓑ symptoms of some conditions change over time.

- Ⓒ other diseases can mimic fibromyalgia symptoms.

- Ⓓ a diagnosis can be missed if a patient has many symptoms.

14 In Des Quinn's response to the study, he says that

- Ⓐ this research is likely to be closely scrutinised.

- Ⓑ the findings should be treated with caution.

- Ⓒ the researchers make unsubstantiated claims.

- Ⓓ the results are a reproduction of previous findings.

Text 2: Antibiotic prescriptions

'The antibiotic crisis has come,' says Chris Del Mar, Professor of Public Health at Bond University on the Gold Coast, Australia. 'We are getting reports from all around the world of multi-resistant organisms; resistant to every antibiotic we know.' The consequences of this development could be catastrophic. 'It could mean a return to the pre-antibiotic era, when people died of pneumonia,' Del Mar says. 'As well as direct deaths from antibiotic resistance, you'd also have the inability to use antibiotic cover for high-risk procedures, which we now take as standard care. That includes things like joint replacements, for example. So that means a lot of orthopaedic surgery would be too dangerous to do.'

One approach to tackling this crisis is to reduce unnecessary antibiotic prescriptions across hospitals and primary care. In Australia, a 2016 report found that family doctors generate 88% of antibiotic prescriptions. According to Del Mar, these rates of over-prescribing emerged from a widespread **better safe than sorry approach** from earlier days in primary care when resistance wasn't so problematic. Consequently, patients have come to expect antibiotic prescriptions when they visit their family doctor. 'An unwritten bond has been built up between doctor and patient in Australia that's led to a dizzying spiral of increasing antibiotic use' says Professor John Turnidge, program lead for the Australian Commission on Safety and Quality in Health Care's (ACSQHC) National Antimicrobial Utilisation Surveillance Program.

Turnidge believes another reason for high rates of antibiotic-prescribing is a fear of losing patients. 'General practice is a private business and you've got to keep your customer satisfied, so to speak. There's always a concern that if you don't write the prescription, the patient will go to the family doctor down the road or to the 24-hour clinic to get it.' This problem may be alleviated somewhat in Australia if patients were required to register at a single general practice clinic rather than being able to freely move from one to another. Such a restriction would leave doctors less pressured to placate them.

While there are obviously cases in which antibiotic prescriptions are well-warranted, recent research has also shown that doctors considered as 'cautious' prescribers actually have the same rate of adverse outcomes from infections as 'enthusiastic' prescribers. 'I think this suggests that family doctors who are cautious prescribers still give antibiotics where they are needed. The difference lies in the larger numbers of people who probably don't need the antibiotics.' says Dr Justin Coleman, Chair of NPS MedicineWise's 'Choosing Wisely Australia' initiative. 'And that's really where we need to make the changes.'

What can family doctors do? One approach is to intervene at the prescribing stage. 'Delayed prescribing' is a strategy in which a prescription, or 'script', is written for antibiotics, but the patient is asked not to fill it for 48 hours. 'It does work in the sense that only a third of patients are ever likely to fill the script,' says Turnidge. 'But the irony of that is if you need an antibiotic, you actually need it now. Waiting two days isn't a great idea.' Turnidge does, however, suggest that delayed prescribing is useful as a deflection strategy because it sends the message to patients that says, 'No, you don't need antibiotics now.' Another strategy being considered by the ACSQHC is introducing scripts that expire within two weeks of being written. Turnidge believes **this** could be very effective because it will prevent patients from storing prescriptions for weeks or months then using it for some other indication.

A third strategy is providing patient education within the consultation. 'It is about having that conversation with the patient at the time, getting them to understand that antibiotics are actually rather precious things and should only be prescribed when doctors really think the patient is likely to benefit,' Turnidge says. Del Mar seemingly agrees and adds, 'It's also important to personalise the message of antibiotic resistance for the individual. I tell patients that if you take antibiotics and then subsequently get an infection like meningitis or pneumonia, it can be very difficult to get on top of the serious infection if there's a resistant strain involved.'

In reality, however, family doctors are busy. The option of simply giving the patient what they want can still seem a lot easier than explaining why the prescription can't be provided, particularly when there is a waiting room full of people. Del Mar believes that doctors need to be able to inform patients about the safe and effective use of antibiotics, but in a way that won't make the consultation any longer. Posters and leaflets could be given to doctors to help communicate the information quickly and clearly. Turnidge agrees with this objective, and says that the use of instructional aids could help doctors convey the right message in a timely way.

Text 2: Questions 15–22

15 In the first paragraph, the writer uses quotes from Professor Chris Del Mar

(A) to illustrate some potential outcomes of increasing antibiotic resistance.

(B) to highlight how undergoing surgery is already risky due to antibiotic resistance.

(C) to clarify some misunderstandings about antibiotic resistance.

(D) to establish the main causes of antibiotic resistance.

16 What is meant by the '**better safe than sorry approach**'?

(A) Patients went to family doctors rather than hospitals for their antibiotics.

(B) Patients started to become aware of how dangerous the antibiotic resistance problem is.

(C) Increasing antibiotic resistance was a deterrent to over-prescription by family doctors.

(D) Family doctors tended to prescribe antibiotics as a precautionary measure.

17 Which solution to the problem of overprescribing antibiotics is discussed in the third paragraph?

(A) Removing the right of patients to attend a number of different clinics.

(B) Abolishing clinics which are open all-hours.

(C) Offering support to clinics with fluctuating patient numbers.

(D) Withdrawing the financial incentive to prescribe antibiotics.

18 What point does Dr Justin Coleman make about 'cautious' prescribers?

(A) They are solely motivated by concerns about antibiotic resistance.

(B) They see a lower number of adverse outcomes than 'enthusiastic' prescribers.

(C) They care for patients as effectively as 'enthusiastic' prescribers.

(D) They have made active changes to their prescribing habits.

19 What downside of 'delayed prescribing' is mentioned in the fifth paragraph?

(A) Doctors are uncomfortable telling patients that they can't have the antibiotics now.

(B) It might be unsafe to make patients wait two days before taking antibiotics.

(C) Patients don't like being asked to wait two days before taking antibiotics.

(D) Two thirds of patients will never fill the prescription for antibiotics.

20 What does the word '**this**' in the fifth paragraph refer to?

(A) making patients wait before receiving a script

(B) reducing the waiting time before scripts can be filled

(C) limiting the number of prescriptions per patient

(D) giving patients scripts that are valid for a limited period of time

21 According to Professor Del Mar, patient education should

(A) highlight the individual's role in adding to the antibiotic crisis.

(B) occur when the doctor thinks it will be advantageous to the patient.

(C) be tailored to suit the patient's own circumstances.

(D) include sufficient information for the patient to make the right choice.

22 What goal does Del Mar share with Turnidge in the final paragraph?

(A) to create longer standard appointment times so that family doctors are not rushed

(B) to give family doctors the tools they need to educate patients more efficiently

(C) to familiarise patients with the prescription writing process so that they know what to expect

(D) to ensure that written information about antibiotic over-prescription is sent to all patients

TIME ALLOWED: **READING TIME:**   **5 MINUTES**
                             WRITING TIME: **40 MINUTES**

Read the case notes and complete the writing task which follows.

Notes:

Assume that today's date is 4 July 2020.
You are a hospital doctor on a geriatric ward and an elderly patient is now ready for discharge.

PATIENT DETAILS

Name:	Mr John Beattie
DOB:	23 March 1930 (90 y.o.)
Address:	20 New Street, Newtown

Social Background:	Labourer (retired)
	Widowed (wife died 2 yrs ago), now lives alone
	2 sons: Bob, 46 y.o. – lives 500 km away, w 2 children
	Sean, 42 y.o. – divorced, lives 10 km away, has M.S.
	(walks w cane – wheelchair used sometimes)
	Care-giver visits 3x/wk (help w ADLs)
	Cleaner visits 1x/wk
	Interests: watching sport on TV (partic. football)

Allergies:	Peanuts
Family History:	Nil

Past medical history:	1982: hypertension
	2008: osteoarthritis R hip
	2010: osteoarthritis both knees
	2015: coronary artery disease (CAD)

Current medications:	Enalapril 1x/day (hypertension)
	Paracetamol 2x/day (osteoarthritis)
	ACE inhibitor (benazepril) 30 mg/day (CAD)

Hospital treatment record:

1 July 2020	Admission to ED
	<u>Subjective</u>: pain (7/10) L side, (fall in kitchen, found on floor by care-giver)
	<u>Objective</u>: BP normal (120/80), pulse 78 bpm, BMP (basic metabolic panel) normal
	Height: 163cm, Weight: 75kg, BMI: 28 (healthy)
	<u>Diagnosis</u>: minor trauma (bruising) L hip & L arm, laceration above L eye
	Hip/arm fractures ruled out – plain X-rays
	No sutures required, current meds continued

2 July 2020	Transfer to geriatric ward
	Recovering well
	<u>Discussion w pt</u>: wishes to live w either son (lost confidence living alone)
3 July 2020	<u>Discussion w sons</u>:
	Father = ↑fall risk → ?care home
	Bob: cannot care for father (distance & children), suggests local care home for immediate care (long-term residential solution to be arranged later)
	Sean: wants to care – prevented by MS, eventually agrees to care home
4 July 2020	Pt agrees to care home
	<u>Immediate care plan</u>:
	Monitor medication compliance
	Wash laceration w soap & water only (to stop infection)
	Hospital physiotherapist to visit 2x/wk (provide exercises ↑ROM L hip & arm)
	Note: geriatric ward outpatient clinic appt. 15 July, transport to be arranged by care home staff
Plan:	Write to manager of care home

Writing Task:

Using the information in the case notes, write a transfer letter to Ms Keller, Care Home Manager, outlining Mr Beattie's relevant medical history, hospital treatment and ongoing care needs. Address the letter to Ms Barbara Keller, Manager, Green Acres Care Home, 200 Green Street, Newtown.

In your answer:

- **Expand the relevant notes into complete sentences**
- **Do <u>not</u> use note form**
- **Use letter format**

The body of the letter should be approximately 180–200 words.

Part A

In this part of the test, you'll hear two different extracts. In each extract, a health professional is talking to a patient.

For **questions 1–24**, complete the notes with information you hear.

Now, look at the notes for extract one.

Extract 1: Questions 1–12

You hear a consultant hand surgeon talking to a patient called Sarah Day. For **questions 1–12**, complete the notes with a word or short phrase that you hear.

You now have thirty seconds to look at the notes.

Patient: Sarah Day

Onset of condition (one year ago)

- (1) _____ sensation in right thumb, index and middle finger
- thumb becomes (2) _____ and difficult to use
- accompanying pain compared to (3) _____
  - radiating to lower arm
  - most noticeable when she needs to (4) _____ objects
- affecting work as a shop fitter – now unable to do tasks such as (5) _____

Initial diagnosis and treatment

- provisional diagnosis of (6) _____
- gained some relief by using **a** (7) _____ and ice packs
- prescribed (8) _____ (no longer effective)
- referral to physiotherapist
  - recommended wrist exercises and (9) _____ (ineffective)

Medical and family background

- **(10)** _____ to right wrist (four years ago)
- episodes of insomnia (past five years)
  - since death of mother from **(11)** _____
- keen to discuss details of **(12)** _____

Extract 2: Questions 13–24

You hear an orthopaedic surgeon talking to a patient called Bryan Rigby. For **questions 13–24**, complete the notes with a word or short phrase that you hear.

You now have thirty seconds to look at the notes.

Patient: Bryan Rigby

Onset of Symptoms (three years ago):

- pain in left knee, described as **(13)** _____ and fairly constant
- bouts of more severe pain linked to **(14)** _____ or application of pressure
- knee feels hot to the touch
- appears **(15)** _____ (compared to right knee)
- reports no trauma
- possible link to work as **(16)** _____

Triggers:
- long periods kneeling on a hard floor – no **(17)** _____
- frequently uses **(18)** _____ (exacerbates symptoms)
- certain tasks at work – e.g. **(19)** _____ at an exhibition
- gardening – e.g. **(20)** _____ – even for short periods

Treatment:
- investigations ruled out **(21)** _____
- provisional diagnosis of bursitis
  - management of symptoms with analgesia
- **(22)** _____ X-ray (results inconclusive)
- asks about the possibility of **(23)** _____ in the future
  - concerned about risk of permanent damage
  - mentions family history of **(24)** _____

Part B

In this part of the test, you'll hear six different extracts. In each extract, you'll hear people talking in a different healthcare setting.

For **questions 25–30**, choose the answer (**A, B** or **C**) which fits best according to what you hear. You'll have time to read each question before you listen. Complete your answers as you listen.

Ⓐ
Ⓑ
Ⓒ

Now look at question 25.

Fill the circle in completely. Example:

---

25 You hear a dentist talking to a patient about dental implants.

What is the patient most concerned about?

Ⓐ the length of recovery time

Ⓑ the number of visits required

Ⓒ the pain involved in the procedure

26 You hear a senior hospital nurse briefing ward staff about patient safety.

What is she doing?

Ⓐ trying to find out how an error occurred

Ⓑ telling them about a complaint she's received

Ⓒ highlighting the importance of working as a team

27 You hear a physiotherapist talking to a patient with a torn ligament.

The patient is having most trouble with

(A) walking uphill.

(B) doing housework.

(C) carrying heavy objects.

28 You hear two community nurses talking about a patient in their care.

They agree that the patient

(A) is in need of a full assessment.

(B) is showing several signs of depression.

(C) is recovering rather slowly after an illness.

29 You hear a dietician talking to a new member of his team.

He's stressing the need to

(A) be sympathetic to patients who are obese.

(B) motivate patients to lose weight before surgery.

(C) make patients aware of the need to attend all sessions.

30 You hear two hospital nurses talking about a patient.

What do they decide about him?

(A) He's ready for discharge.

(B) He needs to have more privacy.

(C) He should be moved within the ward.

Part C

In this part of the test, you'll hear two different extracts. In each extract, you'll hear health professionals talking about aspects of their work.

For **questions 31–42**, choose the answer (**A, B** or **C**) which fits best according to what you hear. Complete your answers as you listen.

Now look at extract one.

Fill the circle in completely. Example:

Ⓐ
Ⓑ
Ⓒ

Extract 1: Questions 31–36

You hear a psychiatric nurse called Marcus Enright giving a presentation on the subject of psychiatric hospitals.

You now have 90 seconds to read **questions 31–36**.

31   What concern does Marcus have about what are called 'sectioned' patients?

Ⓐ   the physical conditions under which they receive treatment

Ⓑ   the lack of information about their experiences after admission

Ⓒ   the danger they're perceived as posing to the wider community

32   Marcus refers to the 'escape' siren at Broadmoor Hospital in order to illustrate

Ⓐ   how impressive systems are needed to protect the public.

Ⓑ   how easily gossip and excitement can be provoked.

Ⓒ   how anxiety about mental illness is intensified.

33   Marcus suggests that musicians were reluctant to work at a party for patients in the hospital because they

Ⓐ   felt nervous about the lack of security.

Ⓑ   had a rather prejudiced view of the institution.

Ⓒ   were unable to reach agreement on certain issues.

34 Marcus hopes that by creating a podcast, he'll enable patients to

(A) suggest improvements in mental healthcare.

(B) gain confidence by supporting each other.

(C) raise public awareness of their condition.

35 The process of making the podcast has helped Marcus to realise that

(A) society has a limited understanding of certain types of mental illness.

(B) living in secure care can be more frightening than imprisonment.

(C) people are interested in learning more about certain conditions.

36 Marcus hopes that in the future, there will be an increase in

(A) public appreciation of psychiatric hospitals.

(B) documentary films about psychiatric illnesses.

(C) progressive treatment of psychiatric conditions.

Now look at extract two.

Extract 2: Questions 37–42

You hear an interview with a senior respiratory nurse called Joanna Parker, who's talking about a new project for patients with idiopathic pulmonary fibrosis (IPF).

You now have 90 seconds to read questions **37–42**.

37   Joanna says that the main aim of the IPF project was to

   (A)   make patient journey times shorter.

   (B)   provide better quality transport for patients.

   (C)   support patients on their way to and from centres.

38   Joanna says that the project involves

   (A)   persuading nurses to develop professionally.

   (B)   encouraging colleagues to adjust their career path.

   (C)   providing opportunities to learn from experienced staff.

39   Which aspect of the project does Joanna find most surprising?

   (A)   improvements in compliance with treatment

   (B)   the rapid uptake of the new services on offer

   (C)   more consistent access to expert care

40 What does Joanna suggest as a downside of the project?

(A) It's unable to provide round-the-clock assistance.

(B) It may be unsuitable for the hearing impaired.

(C) There's no face-to-face contact with staff.

41 What is Joanna most enthusiastic about doing in future?

(A) introducing a more inclusive treatment system

(B) improving IPF management procedures

(C) developing existing service centres

42 Joanna advises anyone thinking about setting up a similar project to ensure that

(A) staff have clear procedures to follow.

(B) nurses' job satisfaction is a high priority.

(C) cases are processed as quickly as possible.

OET SAMPLE TEST

ROLEPLAYER CARD NO. 1	**MEDICINE**

SETTING	Doctor's Clinic
PATIENT	You are 32 years old and were diagnosed with adult-onset asthma one year ago. Dust mites are a major trigger for your asthma. Today you are seeing your doctor for your annual asthma review.
TASK	• When asked, say you've been waking up coughing and wheezing. You've just stopped playing sport because it makes you wheeze, and you sometimes feel short of breath during the day.
	• When asked, say you think you've reduced your exposure to dust mites in your home because you now use allergy covers on your mattress, you removed the carpets, and you regularly wipe down surfaces.
	• When asked, say you finished your preventer medication a few months ago and haven't bought a replacement. You use your reliever when you have symptoms, which helps a little bit.
	• Say the preventer inhaler didn't seem to help you very much, so you don't think you need to start using it again.
	• Say you didn't realise there were risks to using the reliever inhaler frequently. You'll follow the advice and buy a new preventer inhaler.
	• Say you'll come back in four weeks.

       SAMPLE TEST

OET SAMPLE TEST

CANDIDATE CARD NO. 1	**MEDICINE**

SETTING	Doctor's Clinic
DOCTOR	This 32-year-old patient was diagnosed with adult-onset asthma one year ago. Dust mites were identified as a major trigger. You are seeing the patient for his/her annual asthma review.
TASK	• Find out about patient's asthma symptoms (e.g., any change, effect on daily activities/sleep, etc.).
	• Review patient's asthma triggers (e.g., exposure to dust mites, any control measures tried, etc.).
	• Explore patient's asthma self-management strategies (e.g., daily use of inhaled corticosteroid preventer, frequency of salbutamol reliever use, etc.).
	• Explain risks of overusing salbutamol reliever (e.g., increased airway hyper-responsiveness, uncontrolled asthma, asthma-related hospital admission more likely, etc.). Advise patient to purchase replacement preventer.
	• Emphasise importance of using preventer daily (e.g., reduced swelling/inflammation in airways, lowered sensitivity to triggers, decreased mucus production, etc.).
	• Recommend follow-up appointment in four weeks (e.g., monitor treatment effect, review medication, etc.).

       SAMPLE TEST

ROLEPLAYER CARD NO. 2   MEDICINE

SETTING   Doctor's Clinic

PATIENT   You are 45 years old and you are concerned about an unusual mole on your leg. The doctor has just finished examining the mole.

TASK

- When asked, say you first noticed the mole because it started itching about 3 months ago. You think it has grown since then. Sometimes it bleeds a bit.
- When asked, say you like to sunbathe in your rooftop garden. You go on beach holidays whenever you can because you like to work on your tan.
- Say the doctor must be able to tell you if it is skin cancer. You don't want to wait until you have a dermatology appointment.
- Say you've never worried about getting skin cancer before because you're always tanned, and you didn't think you were at risk.
- Say you will definitely stay out of the sun from now on.
- Say you will attend the dermatology appointment once you receive your referral letter.

© Cambridge Boxhill Language Assessment (2022)   SAMPLE TEST

CANDIDATE CARD NO. 2   MEDICINE

SETTING   Doctor's Clinic

DOCTOR   This 45-year-old patient has an atypical mole on his/her leg. You have examined the mole and observe that it is dark brown and asymmetrical with an 8mm diameter and an ill-defined margin. You suspect melanoma.

TASK

- Find out more about patient's mole (e.g., onset, itchiness, enlarging/changing, bleeding, etc.).
- Find out about patient's level of exposure to ultraviolet (UV) light (e.g., sunlight, sunbeds, etc.).
- Explain need for referral to dermatology (e.g., further assessment, biopsy, diagnosis, etc.).
- Resist patient's request for diagnosis (e.g., need for tests, range of possible diagnoses, no benefit in speculation etc.). Reassure patient about waiting time (e.g., appointment within week, diagnosis as soon as possible, etc.).
- Educate patient about skin cancer (e.g., all skin-types prone, UV light cause, especially repeated/sudden/intense UV exposure, etc.). Advise on sun safety (e.g., protective clothing, sunscreen, avoidance of hot sun 10am–4pm, etc.).
- Explain next steps (e.g., wait for referral letter, attend appointment etc.).

© Cambridge Boxhill Language Assessment (2022)   SAMPLE TEST

Blepharitis: Texts

Text A

Epidemiology & causes

Blepharitis is a group of conditions characterised by inflammation of the eyelid margin. It can be divided into anterior blepharitis and posterior blepharitis.

- Blepharitis accounts for at least 5% of ophthalmological presentations in primary care.
- Staphylococcal blepharitis is more common in women, otherwise all forms are equally common in both sexes.
- Blepharitis can occur at all ages but most commonly starts in the fourth and fifth decades of life.
- Staphylococcal infection, seborrhoeic dermatitis, meibomian gland dysfunction, or any combination of these may be a factor in causing blepharitis.

- Blockage of the Meibomian glands means secretions may be deficient or of poor quality resulting in increased tear evaporation and dry eyes (seborrhoeic dermatitis and rosacea also both affect meibomian gland function, and are therefore often associated with blepharitis).
- Demodex mites which infest the eyelid margin may contribute to both anterior and posterior blepharitis. They, their excreta or the body's inflammation response may block follicles and glands.
- Anterior blepharitis can predispose an individual to posterior disease and vice versa.

Text B

Eyes are sore or gritty. There may be itching or burning.

- Eyelids may stick together on waking.
- There may be long periods of exacerbations and remissions.
- Symptoms are worse in the morning.

There may also be symptoms of associated conditions:

- dry eye syndrome: watery eyes, blurred vision, dry eyes, intolerance of contact lenses.

- seborrhoeic dermatitis: dandruff, oily skin, facial rashes.
- rosacea: facial flushing, redness or telangiectasia (dilated/broken blood vessels).

On examination, symptoms may be minimal when compared to the reported severity. Some possible signs are characteristic to each type of blepharitis but may overlap where there is mixed pathology.

Anterior blepharitis	Staphylococcal	Dilated blood vessels around lid margin, crusting around base of lashes (= collarettes), eyelash deformity, depigmentation or loss.
	Seborrhoeic	Skin rash, hyperaemia (increased blood flow) and greasy appearance of anterior lid margin with lashes stuck together. Soft scaling along length of eyelash. Less inflammation. Signs of seborrhoeic dermatitis on scalp, ear or skin folds.
Posterior blepharitis	Meibomian gland dysfunction	Meibomian gland orifices are covered with small oil globules or foam. Glands may be dilated or visibly obstructed. May be telangiectasia and scarring. May be small swelling or lump(s) on the eyelid.

Text C

Diagnosis & Investigations

Lid skin - may be slightly inflamed. Look for concurrent dermatological conditions: scaly or flaking, vesicles, dilated blood vessels or pustules. **Important:** look for associated lesions that may indicate basal cell carcinoma or squamous cell carcinoma.

Lashes - loss frequently occurs in anterior disease and occasionally in long-standing posterior disease. **Be wary of localised lash loss**: sebaceous gland carcinoma may mimic chronic blepharitis - refer if unsure. Look for crusting or hard scales and/or greasiness.

Lid margin - look for inflammation around the meibomian gland orifices or the capping of meibomian gland orifices (looks like a row of yellow droplets along the lid margin).

Tear film - frequently deficient in most forms of blepharitis; may also be foamy.

Conjunctiva - may be infected. Conjunctivitis may be present. Evert eyelid to view tarsal conjunctiva. Scarring can occur in long-standing disease.

Cornea - inferior punctate epithelial erosions, scarring and neovascularisation may all be found in severe forms. Thinning and ulceration are rare but sight-threatening – refer at once.

There are no specific tests: diagnosis is made on examination. Slit-lamp examination is appropriate with severe or resistant symptoms, or with signs of other eye disease. Swabbing may be appropriate in severe or recurrent cases. Biopsy is mandatory in cases where malignancy is suspected (usually - but not exclusively - in the older patient).

Text D

Eyelid hygiene may control simple low-grade blepharitis and should be used regardless of the need for additional treatment. It should be performed twice daily (acute phase) and once at other times.

Action	Method
Warm compresses	Soak a cloth/cotton wool pad with hot water - apply to closed eyes for minimum five (Ideally 10) minutes. Avoid excessive heat
Lid massage (esp for posterior disease)	Massage the closed eyelids in a circular way. Move along length of each lid.
Lid cleansing	Use a cotton bud dipped in cleansing solution, e.g. baby shampoo (diluted 1:10 in warm water), or bicarbonate of soda or soap.

If there is an infection, consider antibiotics:

Topical antibiotics (First line choice)	Dose	Duration
Chloramphenicol ointment (fusidic acid as alternative)	one drop, 3 – 4 x /day (both eyes)	6 weeks

Systemic oral antibiotics e.g.	Dose	Duration
minocycline	50–100 mg 2x/day	6–12 weeks
doxycycline	100 mg 1x /day	
azithromycin	500 mg pd, 3 days pw	3–4 weeks

Avoid oral antibiotic treatment if excessive exposure to the sun is likely (risk of photosensitivity), in pregnancy/ breastfeeding and children under the age of 12 years or in individuals with chronic kidney disease but, if essential, doxycycline is a safer option. Repeated courses may be necessary.

Part A

TIME: 15 minutes

- Look at the four texts, **A–D**, in the separate **Text Booklet** that precedes the questions.
- For each question, **1–20**, look through the texts, **A–D**, to find the relevant information.
- Write your answers on the spaces provided in this **Question Paper**.
- Answer all the questions within the 15-minute time limit.
- Your answers should **only** be taken from texts **A–D** and must be correctly spelt.

Blepharitis: Questions

Questions 1–7

For each question, **1–7**, decide which text (**A**, **B**, **C** or **D**) the information comes from. You may use any letter more than once.

In which text can you find information about

1   the time of day when blepharitis is most symptomatic?   _____

2   preparing materials for cleaning around the eyelids in cases
      of blepharitis?   _____

3   the need to take immediate action if certain symptoms are
      present in part of the eye?   _____

4   the time of life when people are most at risk of developing
      blepharitis?   _____

5   the incidence of blepharitis relative to other eye diseases?   _____

6   people who may react badly to some blepharitis treatments?   _____

7   how to distinguish between different forms of blepharitis?   _____

Questions 8–13

Answer each of the questions, **8–13**, with a word or short phrase from one of the texts. Each answer may include words, numbers or both.

8   What signs of cancer should be checked for when examining eyelid skin for blepharitis?

      _____

9   What can result from persistent cases of blepharitis where conjunctivitis is a factor?

      _____

10   What test is indicated for blepharitis if symptoms are failing to respond to treatment?

      _____

11 Which form of blepharitis can be influenced by a patient's gender?

_____

12 What is the recommended duration of warm compress treatment?

_____

13 How long should a course of topical antibiotics for blepharitis last?

_____

Questions 14–20

Complete each of the sentences, **14–20**, with a word or short phrase from one of the texts. Each answer may include words, numbers or both.

14 If the Meibomian glands are blocked, there is likely to be a rise in

_____ , causing dry eyes.

15 Waste from _____ living in the eye margins may be a factor in blepharitis.

16 Localised loss of lashes can indicate _____ , which closely resembles chronic blepharitis.

17 For blepharitis, the correct dose of Azithromycin is _____ daily, for three days a week.

18 Doxycycline is preferred to other systemic oral antibiotics for patients with

_____ problems.

19 A programme of _____ should always be part of blepharitis treatment.

20 The margin of the anterior eyelid may appear _____ _____ in cases of seborrhoeic anterior blepharitis.

Part B

In this part of the test, there are six short extracts relating to the work of health professionals. For **questions 1–6**, choose the answer (**A**, **B** or **C**) which you think fits best according to the text.

Fill the circle in completely. Example:

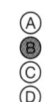

1 The purpose of this guideline on Aseptic Non-Touch Technique is to

(A) introduce a revised classification of items used in invasive procedures.

(B) outline the steps involved in performing a particular type of invasive procedure.

(C) give details of a means of reducing patient risk during invasive procedures.

Aseptic Non-Touch Technique (ANTT)

Protecting key parts

Maintaining asepsis during invasive procedures is a core component of ANTT. Where key parts of equipment become contaminated with pathogenic microorganisms and asepsis is not maintained, there is an increased risk infections to vulnerable patients. Therefore, it is imperative to identify the key parts required for any invasive procedure, in order that they can be protected. Not touching key parts, either directly or indirectly, is critical to achieving asepsis. To identify key parts in any invasive procedure, consider which part(s) of equipment will have direct contact with a susceptible body site or sterile fluids. For example, in intravenous therapy (IV), key parts are those which come into direct contact with the intravenous medication/fluid, such as needles, syringe tips, or catheters that will be used to administer the IV. In wound care, consider all the dressing pack equipment as key parts.

2 The hospital policy on chaperones makes the point that

(A) medical staff must record why they were unwilling to treat a patient without one.

(B) a patient's views on having one can only be ignored in certain circumstances.

(C) there is a degree of flexibility in appointing a suitable person to be one.

Hospital chaperone policy

If any personal care is to be given by a member of the opposite sex, the individual must be offered the option of a chaperone. The chaperone must be acceptable to the person receiving care. Wherever possible, a chaperone should be a healthcare professional, but in cases where such a person is unavailable, and if the examination/procedure cannot be safely postponed, then the patient must be offered the opportunity to invite a relative, carer or friend to be present. If this is not possible, then a non-clinical member of staff from the healthcare team may be asked to undertake the function. If the patient declines the offer of a chaperone during a procedure, this should be respected. If the healthcare professional does not want to proceed with care when the patient has refused a chaperone, the reasons must be explained to the patient.

3 The regulations on cleaning medical devices remind the reader that

(A) cleaning should where possible be performed by the relevant specialist departments.

(B) it may sometimes be necessary to prove that correct procedures have taken place.

(C) a new system for recording the use of such equipment has been implemented.

Cleaning and decontamination of medical devices

Guidance on the prevention of Creutzfeldt-Jakob disease (CJD) or variant Creutzfeldt-Jakob disease (vCJD) means that special consideration must be given to the use and decontamination of any devices which are likely to become contaminated with high risk matter.

The Infection Prevention and Control (IPC) Team and Sterile Services can provide support, but departments likely to encounter tissue or medical devices which may become contaminated with CJD/vCJD proteins must have a written procedure for dealing with such devices.

Wherever it is necessary to quarantine instruments or other reusable medical devices prior to cleaning, it is essential to discuss this with the relevant reprocessing area and also the Surgical Instrument Manager (or their appointed deputy), who will act as the Responsible Person and ensure that all relevant steps are followed and that any relevant documentation is retained for any future inspection.

---

4 The guidelines on caring for patients with transmissible infections mention the need to

(A) organise the schedules of relevant staff in a certain way.

(B) cancel any transfers that have previously been planned for them.

(C) take specific precautions when carrying out their treatment.

Care of patients in isolation with transmissible infections

It is preferable that a designated nurse is assigned to the patient on each shift, in order to reduce the risk of cross-infection. Where this is not possible, any procedures necessary for this patient, e.g. dressing changes, should be performed following the completion of all other duties. Medical staff and associated healthcare professionals, including those conducting ward rounds, should also ensure that patients in isolation are seen last. If a patient in isolation must be moved out of their room, an assessment of the clinical need for, and risk of, such a movement should be carried out by the affected staff. For emergency advice outside normal working hours, the on-call medical microbiologist can be contacted via the main switchboard.

5 This memo states that when controlled drugs are required, staff must

(A) verify each stage of the delivery journey from pharmacy to patient.

(B) avoid trying to obtain them in person unless absolutely necessary.

(C) follow new procedures to ensure that the correct drugs reach the correct patient.

To:	All staff
Subject:	Transport of controlled drugs

All controlled drugs (CDs) ordered in the morning will be signed out by the pharmacy porter and delivered to the relevant department in a sealed purple bag. On receipt, the registrant should check that the seal number and the patient number or name on the bag matches that in the porter's records. Finally, they should also check that the drug delivered matches the request made, before signing to acknowledge receipt of the purple bag. Should the CDs be needed urgently, they may instead be collected from the pharmacy by the registrant. It is imperative that valid identification is shown in such circumstances. This person will sign the received section of the CD requisition form as well as the Pharmacy electronic signature pad, which inserts the signature onto the CD register.

6 The extract from a policy document includes information on

(A) the means by which staff should obtain PPE when needed.

(B) the procedure for staff who need to raise any issues with PPE.

(C) the requirement for staff to regularly study PPE regulations.

Use of hospital personal protective equipment

All employees are responsible for using hospital provided personal protective equipment (PPE) (including any respiratory protective equipment (RPE)) in the way that it is intended to be used, as they have been instructed and in accordance with the manufacturer's instructions. When not in use, PPE should be stored in the facilities provided. Staff are required to practise a high standard of hygiene and make proper use of the facilities provided for washing, showering or bathing, therefore any PPE which could cause contamination must be removed for cleaning/disposal before eating and drinking. Defects or potential risks to health and safety identified in any of the above, including in defined methods of work, devices or facilities, or any item of PPE (including RPE) must be reported promptly to the designated responsible person (e.g. department manager or supervisor)

In this part of the test, there are two texts about different aspects of healthcare. For **questions 7–22**, choose the answer (**A**, **B**, **C** or **D**) which you think fits best according to the text.

Fill the circle in completely. Example:

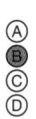

Text 1: The treatment of phantom limb pain using virtual reality

Following amputation, the patient commonly experiences the amputated limb as still intact. This so-called phantom limb can sometimes be painful – something which can have far-reaching implications for the patient's life. For instance, psychological adjustment to amputation is negatively correlated with levels of phantom limb pain (PLP) and amputees with PLP are less likely to use a prosthetic limb. This in turn often results in the restriction of normal activities and is associated with higher levels of depression.

One promising development in the treatment of PLP for amputees is a device known as a mirror box which allows an amputee to view a reflection of their surviving arm or leg in the space that their phantom limb would occupy. For some patients, this can induce vivid sensations of movement which appear to originate from the muscles and joints of their phantom arm as well as reduce PLP. It does, however, require the patient to remain in a fairly fixed position in order to see the mirror. It also depends on patients maintaining focus on the image of the phantom limb and ignoring their intact limb (which provides the movement of the phantom limb via its reflection).

A new approach to PLP uses an immersive virtual reality (IVR) headset and sensors rather than mirrors to create a full body image of the patient with all limbs intact. In our study, participants used this system for 30-minute sessions to complete four tasks. These involved using the virtual limb to touch coloured tiles which light up, hit or kick a virtual ball, track the motion of a moving virtual stimulus, and direct a virtual stimulus towards a target. IVR gives a similar illusion to the mirror box but when using it, only the virtual phantom limb moves – the illusion is unconnected to the patient's position or orientation.

Our first participant was PK, a 63-year-old male left upper-limb amputee. PK suffered with severe PLP 'twenty-four seven'. He described his phantom arm as being shorter than his remaining arm, with the elbow constantly bent at a right angle and with the fingers in a cupped position. PK suffered with intense flashes of immobilising pain in this phantom limb. WW, our second patient, was a 60-year-old male right lower-limb amputee who wore a prosthetic leg. His phantom pain was less severe than that of PK, but he reported that: 'it's always there, like a nagging sensation'. The most distressing part of his condition was sudden bursts of severe pain in the sole of the phantom foot which varied in frequency and interfered with his sleep and his everyday life.

During each session PK reported a decrease in his phantom limb pain, although it returned within a few hours. During his third session, PK reported that 'I actually felt as if it was my left arm that was doing the work. My actual phantom arm … and that was **more like reality than virtual reality**.' He commented that if he could harness the movement in his phantom limb maybe he 'could open [his] fingers and ease the cramping pain a little'. After this session, his pain diary showed an average rating of 6.8 (out of 10) for three days, increasing to an average of 8.3 for the subsequent three days. This is a promising result, given the relatively low frequency of testing sessions.

WW's results were more variable. There were no consistent alterations in pain ratings after the first two sessions, although it should be noted that simulator sickness led the first session to be terminated early. During the second session, his anatomical left leg collided with his stationary prosthetic leg, leading him to comment that this was an 'uneasy sensation' In the third session, however, he removed his prosthesis and, consequently, he was more engaged, he reported no feelings of nausea, and, interestingly, his pain rating at the end of this session showed a decrease from a seven to a three. He also commented that 'It feels as though I'm doing something with my right (phantom) leg.'

Both participants referred to a transferral of sensations into the muscles and joints of the phantom limb. PK supports this more vividly than WW which may indicate the system could potentially benefit upper-limb more than lower-limb amputees – perhaps because of the larger degree of movement afforded by the virtual hand over the virtual foot (i.e., all the fingers move separately whilst for the foot there are no toes – it is represented as wearing a shoe). For the moment, however, **this** remains a tentative possibility.

Both participants reported decreased phantom pain during at least one session. Another common factor is that they both commented on how focused they were on the tasks. This demonstrates the need for control trials to assess the efficacy of this system over and above any pain relief caused purely by the novelty of the tasks and the concentration required. At the same time, it must be established whether a more intense intervention is warranted, since patients' interim pain diaries suggest. the effect of the sessions only lasts for a day or two

Text 1: Questions 7–14

7 What is the writer doing in the first paragraph?

(A) detailing the physical effects of phantom limb pain

(B) describing the impact of phantom limb pain on mental health

(C) outlining the relative incidence of cases of phantom limb pain

(D) explaining the relationship between phantom limb pain and general health

8 What drawback of the mirror box method does the writer mention in the second paragraph?

(A) It may sometimes over-stimulate the user.

(B) It can cause the user unnecessary discomfort.

(C) It relies on the user's ability to concentrate.

(D) It gives the user limited control over their treatment.

9   In the third paragraph, we learn that the VR method of treating phantom limb pain

Ⓐ   requires users to complete an innovative range of tasks.

Ⓑ   works independently of the actions of the remaining limb.

Ⓒ   allows users a lot of freedom in terms of where they undergo it.

Ⓓ   enables patients to achieve results in comparatively little time.

10   In the fourth paragraph, the writer says that the patients called PK and WW

Ⓐ   report experiencing PLP with similar characteristics.

Ⓑ   are affected by in the same way in their daily lives.

Ⓒ   disagree over the most negative aspect of their condition.

Ⓓ   have differing perceptions of the appearance of their phantom limb.

11   When discussing his VR treatment, the patient called PK uses the expression '**more like reality than virtual reality**' in order to

Ⓐ   stress the contribution of VR treatment to reducing his discomfort.

Ⓑ   underline the high degree of physical effort involved in it.

Ⓒ   emphasise the increased optimism he felt after undergoing it.

Ⓓ   highlight the potential control it was giving him over his symptoms.

12   What does the writer suggest about WW's results?

Ⓐ   They confirm the overall efficacy of the treatment method.

Ⓑ   They were influenced by personal issues unrelated to the treatment.

Ⓒ   They represent a misleading picture of the overall value of the treatment.

Ⓓ   They raise a practical question about preparing a patient for treatment.

13 What does 'this' refer to in the seventh paragraph?

(A) a transferral of sensations

(B) a system

(C) a potential benefit

(D) a larger degree of movement

14 One reason the writer thinks that more research into VR treatment is required is that

(A) current results still lack any real consistency.

(B) successes may be due to factors unrelated to it.

(C) comparisons need to be made with other treatment methods.

(D) it is unclear whether improvements result from the treatment itself.

Text 2: The need for a different approach to mental health

It sometimes seems that not a week goes by without a news story featuring a public figure disclosing an ongoing battle with depression. Perhaps the frequency of these revelations should not be a surprise given the apparent ubiquity of feelings of sadness. So, why is it the case that depression is often depicted as such a mystery?

One way to unravel this matter is by telling the stories of some of the patients that I have treated in my psychiatric practice. Kate sought my help when she was unable to complete her PhD thesis. Her distress was compounded by family members telling her to simply 'get on with it'. Jennie, a widow in her 70s, had lost so much weight that her medical specialist suspected cancer, yet tests revealed no physical condition whatsoever. Finally, Simon, a middle-aged professional recently returned from overseas, could not overcome jetlag and lethargy, made worse by bronchitis. He felt utterly defeated. In all these cases, it was clear that their mood had plummeted. Put simply, they, like so many others, all suffered from 'depression', but differed fundamentally in terms of the treatment they required.

Let's return to Kate and her problem in completing her PhD. Having gained an appreciation of her plight, I recommended we explore what might be impeding her. It soon emerged that she couldn't recall ever having received affection from her father, for whom the only thing that mattered in life was material success. He was raised in an impoverished home and, by sheer determination, became a wealthy businessman. Rightly or wrongly, Kate soon came to believe that her ambitious academic pursuit was not only ill-conceived but also not in accord with what her 'authentic' self truly valued – a loving family in which her hoped-for children would flourish.

A physician colleague, stumped by Jennie's severe loss of weight, sought my opinion about her mental state. Her two daughters enabled me to understand the nature of Jennie's malady. They told of their mother's deep sense of loss after her husband's death two years earlier. Grief had assumed a malignant form, escalating into a typical 'retarded depression', which when coupled with her precarious physical condition made electroconvulsive therapy (ECT), administered cautiously and safely, the approach of choice. A short two-week course helped Jennie to make a remarkable recovery. She re-established affectionate relationships with family and friends and was able to reminisce about her 'wonderful marriage'.

I know Simon only too well. His wife urgently sought help from a psychiatrist friend who immediately offered unconditional support to the whole family as well as prescribing antidepressant medication (and an antibiotic for the bronchitis). Although it seemed quite an involved case, he was confident Simon would improve once the medications had kicked in. His prediction was spot on. The patient recovered both physically and psychologically within a few weeks. Simon was in fact me! Although I'd not previously undergone such a terrible experience, I now know that despite appearances, it all came down to nothing more than being exquisitely sensitive to the effects of jetlag. Sometimes it's that straightforward.

Two pivotal lessons arise from my involvement with these patients (and with dozens of others over four decades of psychiatric practice). As Maimonides, the illustrious 12th-century physician, stresses: 'First and foremost, consider the person and only then the symptoms.' And so it should always be the case with what we call depression. We don't catch it as if it were a virus going around. On the contrary, we feel downcast in a particular context. A mental health professional therefore has a role to respond empathically to, and in partnership with, a patient in seeking to understand why he or she presents currently with a particular clinical picture. Only then can the requisite treatment be devised. All these patients show **this** clearly.

A second lesson is inextricably linked to the first – medical professionals are inherently obliged to keep abreast of scientific advances in their field. Consensually agreed guidelines inform us not only of the utility of a specific action or procedure but also of how to best apply it. We can then make an informed judgement as to what is in our patients' best interests.

The concept of depression has always been so ill-defined as to be meaningless. There is a danger that more and more people facing the ups and downs it imposes will be **affixed with the label** and prescribed antidepressants inappropriately. We would be wise to adopt a more nuanced position encompassing a spectrum of clinical scenarios, each pointing to a specific set of interventions to achieve the best possible outcome for a vulnerable person.

Text 2: Questions 15–22

15 In the first paragraph, the writer is puzzled by

    (A)   a widespread perception of depression.

    (B)   certain negative attitudes towards depression.

    (C)   the media attention given to cases of depression.

    (D)   some people's need to publicise their depression.

16 When introducing three of his patients, the writer makes the point that depression

    (A)   may be exacerbated by personal pressure from others.

    (B)   often has certain common root causes in different people.

    (C)   is best managed on an individual rather than a generalised basis.

    (D)   is frequently associated with g other medical conditions.

17 The writer concluded that Kate's problem ultimately stemmed from

    (A)   her father's conviction that she lacked the necessary academic skills.

    (B)   a desire for a future based on different principles from those of her father.

    (C)   a subconscious lack of belief in her own academic abilities.

    (D)   the need to gain the approval of her father in terms of career choice.

18 What do we learn about Jennie's case in the fourth paragraph?

    (A)   Her family had encouraged her to seek a solution to her depression.

    (B)   Her depression originated from a medical rather than a psychological issue.

    (C)   Her depression was felt unlikely to respond to conventional psychiatric therapy.

    (D)   Her depression had evolved into a condition requiring a particular type of treatment.

19 In the fifth paragraph, Simon suggests that his own experience

  (A) confirmed a concern he had regarding his lifestyle.

  (B) showed him the importance of prompt action over cases of depression.

  (C) gave him a useful insight into what it is like to be a psychiatric patient.

  (D) demonstrated that apparently complex cases can have relatively simple causes.

20 What does the word '**this**' refer to in the sixth paragraph?

  (A) the need for an understanding of the patient's situation

  (B) the co-operation between patient and heathcare professional

  (C) the condition that the patient initially presents with

  (D) the approach that is used to treat the patient

21 In the seventh paragraph, the writer says that a patient's interests are overall best served by

  (A) a focus on maintaining ethical standards.

  (B) investment in on-going mental health research.

  (C) developing generally accepted principles for care.

  (D) regular studies of new treatment methods.

22 The writer uses the expression '**affixed with the label**' in order to

  (A) suggest that a more precise definition of depression is needed.

  (B) explain why some may receive unsuitable treatments for depression.

  (C) criticise the way that depression is too often overlooked as a health issue.

  (D) underline the complexities sometimes involved in diagnosing depression.

TIME ALLOWED: READING TIME: 5 MINUTES
                WRITING TIME: 40 MINUTES

Read the case notes and complete the writing task which follows.

Notes:

Assume that today's date is 10 November 2019.

You are a family doctor and have been caring for a young patient following his discharge from hospital.

PATIENT DETAILS:

Name:	Andreas Smith (Mr)
DOB:	23 Oct 1991 (29 y.o.)
Address:	Apartment 1 (ground floor), 194 Springhall Parade, Newtown
Social Background:	Lawyer (graduated in Jan 2018)
	Girlfriend of 3 yrs, supportive, visits 2-3x/wk
	Parents, supportive, visit 1x/wk
	Non-smoker
	Alcohol intake approx. 12 units/wk (mainly beer)
	Interests: reading, music, TV
Allergies:	Nil
Family History:	Mother – osteoarthritis
	Father – gout
	Maternal grandmother – bipolar disorder, died 80 y.o. (stroke)
	Maternal grandfather – died 75 y.o. (heart attack)
	Paternal grandmother & grandfather – unknown
Past medical history:	Childhood chickenpox & measles
	1993 hyperopia, glasses given
	2015 L Rotator cuff injury

Hospital treatment record:

16 March 2019:	Arrival at ED
	MVA (motor vehicle accident): neurologic lesion of spinal cord at T12, resulting in paraplegia (wheelchair required)
	Neurogenic bladder – intermittent urinary catheter
	Colostomy for neurogenic bowel → Baclofen pump (change 4x/yr)
	Transfer to general ward for recovery
20 March 2019:	Good progress
	Medications: corticosteroids, NSAIDs, anticonvulsants, mild opioids, antispasmodics, muscle relaxants
	Mild infection at incision site → antibiotics

13 April 2019:	Ready for discharge
	<u>Discharge plan</u>: continue opioids & NSAIDs 2 months (to be reviewed by family doctor)
	OT & physio visits (↑mobility, weight bearing exercises) & wheelchair (unable to ambulate)
	Community Nurse – help w ADLs

General practice appointment record:

12 June 2019:	<u>Medication review</u>
	Pain well managed
	Continue opioids & NSAIDs prn
	Baclofen pump changed
	Pt coping well
	Reviews w dr approx. 1x/month
8 July 2019:	Community transport arranged for appt – pt. refused, parents brought pt & attended appt w him
	Pain well managed
	Note: pt ↑isolated (won't allow girlfriend/friends to visit)
4 August 2019:	Pt missed appt, rescheduled Sept.
6 September 2019:	Telephone consultation (pt request)
	Fear & anxiety at thought of leaving home
8 October 2019:	Missed appt, rescheduled Nov.
10 November 2019:	Missed face-to-face appt – pt admits ↑anxiety at leaving home → panic attack in transit
	Telephone consultation conducted instead
	?<u>diagnosis</u>: agoraphobia (pt. requests referral to psychiatrist, 'I want some social life back')
Plan:	Refer to psychiatrist

Writing Task:

Using the information in the case notes, write a letter of referral to Dr Besson, psychiatrist, outlining your concerns about the patient and requesting definitive diagnosis and further management. Address the letter to Dr Lucy Besson, Psychiatrist, Newtown Hospital, 111 High Street, Newtown.

In your answer:
- **Expand the relevant notes into complete sentences**
- **Do <u>not</u> use note form**
- **Use letter format**

The body of the letter should be approximately 180–200 words.

Part A

In this part of the test, you'll hear two different extracts. In each extract, a health professional is talking to a patient.

For **questions 1–24**, complete the notes with information you hear.

Now, look at the notes for extract one.

Extract 1: Questions 1–12

You hear a gastroenterologist talking to a new patient called Janina Parker. For **questions 1–12**, complete the notes with a word or short phrase that you hear.

You now have 30 seconds to look at the notes.

Patient:	Janina Parker

Onset of symptoms (18 months ago)

- unexplained **(1)** _____
- extreme fatigue and lack of **(2)** _____
- **(3)** _____ alternating with diarrhoea
- loss of appetite and nausea
- stomach **(4)** _____
- bloating

Investigations and diagnosis

- provisional diagnosis of gluten intolerance
  - doctor also suspected **(5)** _____
- **(6)** _____ and endoscopy administered

  positive for immunoglobulin E antibodies
  - damage to the **(7)** _____ of the small intestine
  - biopsy confirmed diagnosis of coeliac disease
- DEXA scan showed low bone density
  - now taking **(8)** _____

Patient concerns

- fears consequences of long-term malnutrition
- reports feeling increasingly **(9)** _____
- suspects her diet is deficient in **(10)** _____
- requests referral to a **(11)** _____
- asks about the possibility of being prescribed **(12)** _____

Extract 2: Questions 13–24

You hear a podiatrist talking to a patient called Derek Hardy. For **questions 13–24**, complete the notes with a word or short phrase that you hear.

You now have thirty seconds to look at the notes.

Patient: Derek Hardy

Background to condition

- diagnosis of diabetes (six years ago)
  - compliant with monitoring
  - reports that blood sugar levels are **(13)** _____
- **(14)** _____ confirmed (nine months ago)
- recent weight gain attributed to:
  - reduced mobility linked to weakness in right foot
  - **(15)** _____ (age related)

Recent foot problems

- small **(16)** _____ on left foot – now resolved
- swelling to right foot
  - linked to **(17)** _____ sustained when out walking
  - on-going infection on **(18)** _____ of the foot

Foot hygiene

- washes daily – reports some difficulty with **(19)** _____
- applies **(20)** _____ after washing
- sees **(21)** _____ regularly
- usually wears **(22)** _____ – less effective later in the day

Current concerns

- asks for advice about use of **(23)** _____
- requests more frequent check-ups
- worried about developing **(24)** _____ in future

Part B

In this part of the test, you'll hear six different extracts. In each extract, you'll hear people talking in a different healthcare setting.

For **questions 25–30**, choose the answer (**A, B** or **C**) which fits best according to what you hear. You'll have time to read each question before you listen. Complete your answers as you listen.

Now look at question 25.

Fill the circle in completely. Example:

25 You hear a senior nurse in a care home for the elderly briefing new members of her team.

   She says that before beginning a patient assessment, team members should

   (A) ensure all necessary records are up to date.

   (B) deal with any potential trip hazards.

   (C) clean up any liquid spillages.

26 You hear a primary-care doctor talking to a patient.

   What concerns the patient most about his headaches?

   (A) They may be a sign of a more serious illness.

   (B) They seem to be exacerbated by both light and motion.

   (C) They could be triggered by certain medications he's taking.

27 You hear two hospital nurses talking about a patient who's recovering from surgery.

What is the priority for the patient this morning?

(A) double-checking his dietary choices

(B) addressing his personal hygiene needs

(C) requesting a reassessment of his analgesia

28 You hear a community pharmacist talking to a patient.

What is the patient he seeking advice about?

(A) the correct way to take his medication

(B) how to relieve the side effects of his medication

(C) whether he should take his medication in another form

29 You hear two hospital nurses conducting a patient handover

Before the patient can be discharged,

(A) a family member needs to be briefed.

(B) support needs to be put in place in her home.

(C) her independence with a mobility aid needs to be confirmed.

30 You hear two emergency department doctors talking about a patient.

What is concerning them most about him?

(A) some abnormal test results

(B) the way he's reacted to some medication

(C) a lack of background information to inform a diagnosis

Part C

In this part of the test, you'll hear two different extracts. In each extract, you'll hear health professionals talking about aspects of their work.

For **questions 31–42**, choose the answer (**A, B** or **C**) which fits best according to what you hear. Complete your answers as you listen.

Now look at extract one.

Fill the circle in completely. Example:

Extract 1: Questions 31–36

You hear an interview with a nurse trainer called Susan Myers, who's talking about the importance of using compassionate communication skills with patients.

You now have 90 seconds to read **questions 31–36**.

31   What led Susan to set up the training initiative to develop these skills was the realisation that

    (A) they can be hard to implement when most needed.

    (B) many nurses admit a lack of confidence in using them.

    (C) a growing range of healthcare settings are demanding them.

32   Susan points out that patients can be impacted by poor communication skills when

    (A) the workload of nurses prevents frequent interaction.

    (B) information passed between nurses becomes inaccurate.

    (C) nurses lose concentration as a result of long working hours.

33   To illustrate her point about breakdowns in communication, Susan gives the example of patients

    (A) being distracted when receiving upsetting news.

    (B) not understanding the use of specialised language.

    (C) being unable to give answers to important questions.

34 Susan feels that the commonest reason for nurses not listening effectively is

    (A) the frustrations involved in dealing with complicated technology.

    (B) an unwillingness to give patients enough time to explain things.

    (C) stress levels arising from their wide range of responsibilities.

35 Susan has found that nurses who practise mindful listening are more likely to

    (A) adopt a personalised approach to patient care.

    (B) unknowingly pass on the skill to other people.

    (C) remain focused on a conversation for longer.

36 What does Susan suggest about facial expressions?

    (A) They can be even more powerful than speech.

    (B) It's almost impossible to avoid making them.

    (C) Even small ones can reveal our true feelings.

Now look at extract two.

Extract 2: Questions 37–42

You hear a urologist called Dr Marius Glover giving a presentation about the diagnosis and treatment of UTIs – urinary tract infections.

You now have 90 seconds to read **questions 37–42**.

37 Dr Glover's main concern about UTIs is that

    (A) patients often fail to seek treatment early enough.

    (B) the bacteria have a hidden defence mechanism.

    (C) they're a recurrent problem for many patients.

38 Dr Glover finds it strange that midstream urine culture testing is still in use because

    (A) it's based on limited and outdated research.

    (B) it can't easily be adapted for specific patient groups.

    (C) it's being investigated following concerns raised by experts.

39 Dr Glover suggests that the urinary dipstick is

    (A) only useful for initial screening purposes.

    (B) a largely inappropriate testing method.

    (C) unable to identify asymptomatic UTIs.

40 Dr Glover suggests that the prescribing of antibiotics for suspected UTIs

   (A)   may not always be appropriate.

   (B)   is something doctors are cautious about.

   (C)   could conceal the true scale of the problem.

41 Dr Glover is optimistic about Professor Malone-Lee's discovery because it

   (A)   works for patients with antimicrobial resistance.

   (B)   has the capacity to permanently eradicate bacteria.

   (C)   stops the mobilisation of bacteria all around the body.

42 Dr Glover says that one advantage of the 'fidget spinner' device is that it

   (A)   prompts flexible prescribing.

   (B)   is straightforward and easy to use.

   (C)   enables matching of antimicrobials to bacteria.

OET SAMPLE TEST

ROLEPLAYER CARD NO. 1	**MEDICINE**

SETTING — Doctor's Clinic

PATIENT — You are 58 years old. You are normally fit and well, but today you are seeing your regular doctor because you've been having bad headaches recently.

TASK
- When asked, say you're worried about the headaches you've been having lately.
- When asked, say you've had three terrible, throbbing headaches in the last three months. The headaches affect the right side of your head and last for about two days. You have to lie down in a dark room because the light hurts your eyes. You get 'black spots' in your vision before a headache. You also feel very tired and your face becomes tingly.
- When asked, say you've been more stressed lately because you have started studying part-time in the evenings as well as continuing your full-time job.
- Say you don't like putting chemicals in your body, so you really don't want to take medication.
- Say you'll follow the advice the doctor has given. Ask if there's anything else you can do.
- Say you'll keep a headache diary and will make a follow-up appointment.

© Cambridge Boxhill Language Assessment (2022)   SAMPLE TEST

OET SAMPLE TEST

CANDIDATE CARD NO. 1	**MEDICINE**

SETTING — Doctor's Clinic

DOCTOR — This 58-year-old is a regular patient of yours and is normally fit and well. Today, the patient has come to talk to you because he/she is worried about the recent headaches he/she has been having.

TASK
- Find out reason for patient's visit.
- Find out more details about patient's headaches (e.g., frequency, duration, location, severity, associated aura, etc.).
- Explore possible triggers (e.g., stress, environmental/behavioural changes, foods/food additives, etc.).
- Give diagnosis of migraines (e.g., abnormal brain activity, commonly stress-triggered, etc.). Explain medication options (e.g., analgesics, triptans, etc.).
- Advise on non-pharmacological management strategies (e.g., relaxation techniques upon onset, minimising stress, avoiding caffeine/chocolate, etc.).
- Recommend keeping headache diary (e.g., triggers, warning signs, patterns, preventive actions, etc.). Suggest follow-up appointment in two months (e.g., review headache diary, reassess treatment, etc.).

© Cambridge Boxhill Language Assessment (2022)   SAMPLE TEST

ROLEPLAYER CARD NO. 2   MEDICINE

SETTING   Doctor's Clinic

PATIENT   You are 19 years old and you have a painful left big toe. The doctor has just finished examining the toe.

TASK
- When asked, say you noticed that your toe was red and sore about two weeks ago. You play football every day and it's now extremely painful when you kick the ball. You haven't tried to treat it.
- When asked, say the only thing you can think of is that you bought some new football boots, which are a bit tight.
- Say you'll treat the toe as advised, but you can't afford to buy more football boots, so you'll have to continue wearing the tight ones.
- Say you'll go back to your old boots again as you still have them and they're more comfortable. Ask how long it will take for the problem to clear up.
- Say you will follow the doctor's advice and will come back in two weeks if your toe is no better.

© Cambridge Boxhill Language Assessment (2022)   SAMPLE TEST

CANDIDATE CARD NO. 2   MEDICINE

SETTING   Doctor's Clinic

DOCTOR   This 19-year-old patient has a painful left big toe. You have just finished examining the toe. You diagnose an ingrown toenail.

TASK
- Find out further details about patient's toe problem (e.g., onset, level of pain, treatment tried, etc.).
- Give diagnosis (e.g., ingrown toenail with inflammation/seropurulent drainage etc.). Outline common causes of ingrown toenail (e.g., improper trimming/tearing off nail, repetitive running/kicking, ill-fitting footwear, etc.). Explore relevance to patient.
- Explain self-care (e.g., daily warm soapy footbath, topical antibiotic ointment, etc.). Recommend appropriate footwear (e.g., replacement of ill-fitting boots, open-toed footwear, when possible, etc.).
- Advise against continued use of ill-fitting footwear (e.g., further trauma to toe, other toes affected, additional foot problems, etc.).
- Give timescale for healing (e.g., 1–2 weeks, depending on patient compliance, etc.). Recommend follow-up appointment in two weeks if no improvement (e.g., reassessment of toe, consideration for gutter splint/surgical therapy, if necessary, etc.).

© Cambridge Boxhill Language Assessment (2022)   SAMPLE TEST

Shingles: Texts

Text A

Presentation

There is usually a prodromal phase with abnormal skin sensations and pain in the affected dermatome (area of skin served by an individual nerve). The pain can be described as burning, stabbing, or throbbing; can be intermittent or constant, and may be so severe that it interferes with sleep and everyday living. Headache, photophobia, malaise, and fever (less common) may also occur as part of the prodromal phase.

Within 2–3 days (more rarely up to 7 days), a rash typically appears in a dermatomal distribution. It starts as maculopapular lesions then develops into clusters of vesicles, with new vesicles continuing to form over 3–5 days. The rash is usually painful, itchy, and/or tingly, and, unlike other rashes, does not cross the midline of the body. The vesicles then burst, releasing varicella-zoster virus, and crust over within 7–10 days, healing within 2–4 weeks.

The location of symptoms depends on the affected nerve: In immunocompetent people, the infection usually occurs on the face and thorax. In immunocompromised people, the lesions can be more widespread and become disseminated over the whole body (disseminated disease).

Text B

Treatment

Prescribe an oral antiviral treatment within 72 hours of rash onset for people with any of the following criteria:

- Immunocompromised (if the level of immunocompromise is not severe, the rash is localized, the person is not systemically unwell, and they can be closely followed up).
- Non-truncal involvement, such as shingles affecting the neck, face (particularly the eyes), limbs, or perineum.
- Moderate or severe rash.

Consider prescribing oral antiviral treatment within 72 hours of rash onset for all people aged over 50 years to reduce the incidence of post-herpetic neuralgia, which is most common in this age group. If it is not possible to initiate treatment within 72 hours, consider starting antiviral treatment up to one week after rash onset, especially if the person is at higher risk of severe shingles or complications.

In the case of pregnant or breastfeeding women, seek specialist advice before prescribing antiviral treatment.

For immunocompetent children with shingles, antiviral treatment is not usually recommended.

Recommended dosages:

	Immunocompetent adults	Immunocompromised adults* N.B. Continue treatment for 2 days after the lesions have crusted.
Aciclovir	800 mg five times a day for 7 days at 4-hourly intervals (doses should be spaced evenly throughout the day).	800 mg five times a day for 7 days.
Famciclovir	500 mg three times a day for 7 days, or 750 mg 1–2 times a day for 7 days.	500 mg three times a day for 10 days.
Valaciclovir	1000 mg three times a day for 7 days.	1000 mg three times a day for 7 days.

*(if not systemically unwell and if rash is localized)

Text C

Complications

Post-herpetic neuralgia (defined as pain persisting for, or appearing more than, 90 days following rash onset) is the most common complication of shingles and is caused by herpes zoster-induced peripheral nerve damage. Studies indicate that there is a demonstrable increase in the rate of post-herpetic neuralgia in patients over 50 years old.

Other, less common, complications of shingles include:

o Skin changes — scarring, changes in pigmentation, and keloid formation may occur after a shingles rash has healed.

o Superinfection of skin lesions — secondary infection of the lesions, usually with staphylococcal or streptococcal bacteria

o Herpes zoster oticus — occurs when the virus infects the facial nerve (cranial nerve VII). It is characterized by lesions in the ear, facial paralysis, and associated hearing and vestibular symptoms.

o Herpes zoster ophthalmicus — occurs when the virus infects the ophthalmic division of the trigeminal nerve. Complications include keratitis, corneal ulceration, conjunctivitis, optic neuritis, retinitis, glaucoma, and blindness if untreated.

o Peripheral motor neuropathy — occurs when the motor component of the nerve is involved, and causes impaired strength in the affected area.

Text D

Pain management

- For adults with mild pain, offer a trial of paracetamol alone or in combination with codeine or a nonsteroidal anti-inflammatory drug (NSAID), such as ibuprofen.

- If this is not effective, or the person presents with severe pain, consider offering amitriptyline (off-label use), duloxetine (off-label use), gabapentin, or pregabalin.

- The choice of drug depends on the relative contraindications, possible drug interactions, and risk of adverse effects for each person.

- Consider oral corticosteroids in combination with antivirals in the first 2 weeks following rash onset in immunocompetent adults with localized shingles if pain is severe.

- Use clinical judgment, taking into account the risks and benefits of corticosteroid therapy for each person.

- Consult a specialist or refer to the pain team if:

  Pain is inadequately controlled by oral analgesia.

  Strong opioids are being considered.

- For children with pain, offer a trial of paracetamol (avoid the use of NSAIDs). If this is not effective, seek specialist advice.

TIME: 15 minutes

- Look at the four texts, **A–D**, in the separate **Text Booklet** that precedes the questions.
- For each question, **1–20**, look through the texts, **A–D**, to find the relevant information.
- Write your answers on the spaces provided in this **Question Paper**.
- Answer all the questions within the 15-minute time limit.
- Your answers should **only** be taken from texts **A–D** and must be correctly spelt.

Shingles: Questions

Questions 1–7

For each question, **1–7**, decide which text (**A**, **B**, **C** or **D**) the information comes from. You may use any letter more than once.

In which text can you find information about

1 selecting drugs to reduce varying levels of discomfort experienced by patients? _____

2 the stages in the progression of shingles? _____

3 other medical issues which can result from shingles? _____

4 discomfort from shingles which affects a patient's quality of life? _____

5 patients who should not generally be given antiviral drugs for shingles? _____

6 how a shingles rash differs from that associated with other conditions? _____

7 possible permanent consequences of shingles? _____

Questions 8–14

Answer each of the questions, **8–14**, with a word or short phrase from one of the texts. Each answer may include words, numbers or both.

8 After what age are people most likely to develop post-herpetic neuralgia?

_____

9 Which complication of shingles may cause deafness?

_____

10 In a patient with a normal immune system, in which area of the body is the shingles rash most likely to appear?

_____

11   What form does the rash take in the initial stages of shingles?

_____

12   What is the maximum length of time that the shingles rash usually takes to heal?

_____

13   What may be prescribed to an adult with a normal immune system for a severe level of pain in the initial 14 days after the rash appears?

_____

14   If a patient takes Famciclovir twice a day, what is the recommended size of each dose?

_____

Questions 15–20

Complete each of the sentences, **15–20**, with a word or short phrase from one of the texts. Each answer may include words, numbers or both.

15   Further advice should be sought before prescribing _____ for pain.

16   If Aciclovir, Famciclovir or Valaciclovir are given to a patient with a weakened immune system, treatment should be extended for an extra _____ once crusting has occurred.

17   If the shingles rash is in a _____ area and the patient is immunocompetent, oral antivirals should be prescribed within 72 hours of onset.

18   The opinion of an expert should be sought when considering antiviral drugs for

_____.

19   If pain continues for more than _____ after the shingles rash first presents, the patient is considered to be suffering from post-herpetic neuralgia.

20   If a patient develops _____ they could lose their sight if they do not receive treatment.

Part B

In this part of the test, there are six short extracts relating to the work of health professionals. For **questions 1–6,** choose the answer (**A**, **B** or **C**) which you think fits best according to the text.

Fill the circle in completely. Example:

---

1 What does the guideline extract tell medical staff about high-sensitivity troponin I and T tests?

(A) why more than 50% of people test positive

(B) which condition they most accurately identify

(C) how the most reliable results can be obtained

High-sensitivity troponin tests

The initial assessment for a person presenting with suspected acute coronary syndrome is a 12-lead resting ECG and two blood tests (four hours apart) for high-sensitivity troponin I or T. High-sensitivity troponin tests are those that can detect cardiac troponin in at least 50% of the reference population.

Troponin tests used for indications other than suspected acute coronary syndrome are likely to be non-specific markers of myocardial damage. These tests are, for example, useful prognostically but not diagnostically in cases of pulmonary embolism (PE). Troponin levels are elevated in up to half of patients who have a moderate to large PE and are associated with clinical deterioration after PE. However, troponin elevations usually resolve within 40 hours following PE, in contrast to the more prolonged elevation after acute myocardial injury. Computed topographic pulmonary angiography (CPTA) is recommended for the specific diagnosis of PE.

---

2 This update to guidance on post-exposure measles prophylaxis advises that

(A) if injection volume is a concern, the MMR vaccine is preferred over IMIg.

(B) the MMR vaccine should no longer be administered to infants.

(C) IMIg may not give sufficient protection to all patients.

Post-exposure prophylaxis for measles

The national advisory committee on vaccination continues to recommend that immunocompetent individuals over six months of age who are exposed to measles and have no contraindications be given measles-mumps-rubella (MMR) vaccine within 72 hours of exposure. Infants younger than six months should be given intramuscular immunoglobulin (IMIg) at a concentration of 0.5 mL/kg, provided injection volume is not a major concern. Infants six to 12 months old who are identified after 72 hours and within six days of measles exposure should receive IMIg (0.5 mL/kg) if injection volume is not a major concern. For patients who are pregnant or immunocompromised, if injection volume is not a concern, IMIg can be provided at a concentration of 0.5 mL/kg, understanding that recipients 30 kg or more will not receive the measles antibody concentrations that are considered to be fully protective.

---

3 This memo is reminding critical care staff of the guidance on

（A） preparing a child for admittance to the unit as a patient.

（B） allowing a child to see an adult patient in the unit.

（C） family members visiting a child who is a patient in the unit.

To:	Critical Care Unit Staff
Subject:	Recent problems with children in the critical care unit.

Following recent problems, staff are reminded that children should always be accompanied by a responsible person aged over 18. It may occasionally be appropriate for older children to approach the patient's bedside unaccompanied, but there should always be an adult in the waiting area to support them and ensure their safety. As the critical care unit is a potentially dangerous place for children, there should be a maximum of 2 children per adult. However, it is important to remember that the bed space should not become overcrowded. Children have a shorter attention span than adults, therefor it may be useful to suggest to the family that there is an additional adult available when the child comes in. They can then support and care for the child in the waiting area whilst the other adult remains with the patient in the critical care unit for a longer period.

4 This memo is encouraging clinical staff to

（A） consult a specialist before prescribing warfarin.

（B） reduce the number of patients who are prescribed warfarin.

（C） help assess adverse reactions in patients who are prescribed warfarin.

To:	All medical staff
Subject:	Warfarin

Only where there is no other anticoagulant option, or where it would be unsafe to use anything else, should patients be discharged on warfarin. For atrial fibrillation (AF), use a direct oral anticoagulant (DOAC) unless contraindicated. Even if the patient is > 120kg, consider a DOAC. Rivaroxaban, which seems least affected by weight, is the preferred option in patients over 120kg up to 150kg. There are extremely limited data over 150kg, but a DOAC could be considered if there has been no thrombotic stroke in the last 3 months. Please refer patients >120 kg to the anticoagulant service so we can check levels in the future. Patients with AF who are admitted on warfarin should be switched to a DOAC unless contraindicated. If a DOAC is thought to be contraindicated, consider low-molecular-weight heparin temporarily or seek advice from a Haemostasis and Thrombosis Consultant or Anticoagulant Pharmacist.

5 This extract from guidelines on tuberculosis states that personal respiratory protection equipment

(A) has limited effectiveness at preventing transmission.

(B) protects others as well as the wearer.

(C) will be tested on a regular basis.

Infection Control Management of Inpatients with Tuberculosis

The hospital's Infection Prevention and Control Team have responsibility for facilitating the testing of all respiratory protection equipment. The term 'personal respiratory protection' refers to any device such as particulate filter masks worn by an individual to protect them from inhaling harmful particles (as opposed to, for example, surgical masks worn to reduce transmission of infection from the wearer to another person). Personal respiratory protection should be regarded as inferior and secondary to other environmental and infection control measures in reducing the risk of tuberculosis transmission. The equipment should meet the standards of the Health and Safety Executive.

---

6 The main purpose of the email about bed safety sides is to

(A) ensure that they are used appropriately and safely.

(B) highlight some recent issues associated with their use.

(C) point out that they are useful for a wide range of patients.

To:	Medical Personnel
Subject:	Bed Safety Rails

Staff are reminded that patients may be at risk of falling from their bed for many reasons including dementia, delirium, visual impairment, recent paralysis, stroke, and effects of medication. The bed safety side is not a form of restraint, nor is it intended to limit freedom of patients by preventing them from leaving their bed voluntarily. Safety sides are not moving and handling aids, as they have not been safety tested for this purpose. Neither are they intended to restrain patients whose condition disposes them to erratic or violent movement.

The use of a bed safety side is associated with a number of direct and indirect risks to patients, such as severe limb damage when limbs become trapped and asphyxiation due to trapping of the head between mattress and safety side. When using a bed safety side, a full risk assessment must be undertaken.

Part C

In this part of the test, there are two texts about different aspects of healthcare. For **questions 7–22,** choose the answer (**A, B, C** or **D**) which you think fits best according to the text.

Fill the circle in completely. Example:

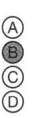

Text 1: Sleep deprivation and malnutrition in hospital

The field of patient safety in hospital has focused on acute adverse events, while regular stressors such as sleep deprivation and malnutrition are unlikely to be detected as preventable adverse events in chart-based studies. In comparison with other patient safety events such as catheter infections, sleep deprivation and malnutrition are less straightforward to quantify, as they are dynamic and occur with varying severity. Even a young, healthy individual will become physiologically stressed and transiently immunocompromised after a **mere** 24 hours of starvation and a poor night's sleep, resulting in acne, fatigue, oral ulcers and impaired judgment—conditions which, in the presence of illness, can worsen or obscure the clinical picture. In frail patients, the effects are magnified further.

The problem of sleep deprivation and malnutrition stressing patients is compounded by the complexity and changes in the way medical care is delivered today, and worsened when hospitals are operating close to full capacity, a trend now widely observed. Consequently, more patients are spending the night in noisy emergency rooms, recovery rooms and even hallways. Over the last decade, emergency room wait times have increased, and more patients spend the night in the recovery room after elective surgery, due to bed shortages. Longer wait lists for procedures require more last-minute rescheduling, stretching the time that patients are without nutrition. Financial pressures have impacted staffing levels and bed flow. Finally, a large number of speciality services results in complex communication layers and communication breakdowns in scheduling inpatient tests and procedures.

Malnutrition affects as many as 30% to 50% of all hospitalised patients. Many are malnourished to begin with due to their illness and multiple comorbidities, and this is easily compounded by wound healing and disruptions in food intake following surgery. A US study showed that only 3% of adult hospital admissions include a diagnosis of malnutrition, suggesting that it remains under-recognised. Furthermore, few patients receive nutritional consults in hospital. Another barrier is the notoriously poor-quality hospital food, consisting of highly processed food from inexpensive suppliers. Hospitals have an opportunity to amend this. Some have taken the lead by serving organic local foods which achieve a broad range of nutritional goals.

In some cases, malnutrition can be stemmed by adopting standardised preoperative protocols. The American Society of Anesthesiologists recommends avoiding extended preoperative fasting and endorses clear liquids up to 2 hours before surgery, but adoption of this practice has been slow. Limiting preoperative fasting is an essential component of Enhanced Recovery after Surgery (ERAS) protocols, which aim to restore physiological function and facilitate recovery. The evidence shows that needless prolongation of fasting after gastrointestinal surgery actually increases the risk of infection and does not reduce the risk of complications such as anastomotic dehiscence. In my workplace, implementing the comprehensive ERAS protocol has led to a significant reduction in postoperative complications and hospital length of stay as well as improving patient satisfaction.

The hospital environment can be noisy, with alarms, phones, hallway conversations and patients sharing rooms. This is then compounded by intercoms, chatter, lights, plus sometimes frequent interruptions at night for medications, vital signs and lab draws. Vital signs may be collected too often and this may actually be detrimental to patients' well-being, as well as representing staff labour that can be diverted from low-risk patients to those at greater risk of physiological collapse. Checks more frequent that the usual (4-hourly) ones could be required to be written deliberately as orders rather than being the **default setting** for some patients. Continuous monitoring via devices that detect patient deterioration may also present a potential solution. Many hospital units, especially intensive care units, continue to use 24-hour lighting, which should be considered a potential source of physiological stress. Hospitals should conduct noise studies, obtain more feedback from patients on the most disruptive sources of noise and aim to mitigate them. There may be even simpler interventions, such as encouraging use of noise-reduction headphones, eye masks, massage and music therapy.

The hospital experience can be dehumanising, and increasing evidence points to the environment as central to quality. An interview study involving 380 discharged patients found that environment was the second-highest predictor of overall satisfaction with care, behind quality of clinical care. Many of the required interventions are easy to implement, low-risk and low-cost, though others will require extensive systems-level planning and careful implementation. The value of rest and nutrition may be underrepresented in the current medical literature. This is a field that may benefit from more interventional research to demonstrate the effectiveness of addressing a patient's basic needs. Nevertheless, hospitals can reduce these physiological stressors by designing more patient-centred hospital systems. As we seek to improve quality through patient-centredness, basic human needs are important in the context of complex medical care. We should view hospitals as healing environments rather than isolated clinical spaces and design patient care accordingly.

Text 1: Questions 7–14

7   The writer suggests that sleep deprivation and malnutrition in hospital are often ignored because

    (A)   they are difficult to measure.

    (B)   little research has been done into them.

    (C)   they mainly affect less vulnerable patients.

    (D)   their consequences are mild.

8.   The word **mere** in the first paragraph is used to emphasise the fact that malnutrition

    (A)   affects patients more quickly when combined with other issues.

    (B)   occurs more rapidly in certain patients.

    (C)   can begin without an obvious cause.

    (D)   causes health issues within a short space of time.

9   What aspect of sleep deprivation and malnutrition is the writer addressing in the second paragraph?

    (A)   the reasons why they can lead to delays in treatment

    (B)   the medical contexts in which most cases are recorded

    (C)   the factors which have led to them becoming more common

    (D)   the fact that they are made more likely by transferring patients

10 In the third paragraph, the writer implies that

(A) patients' diets can deteriorate when they are admitted to hospital.

(B) there is a need for hospitals to share learning on improving nutrition.

(C) hospitals use financial constraints as an excuse for offering inferior food.

(D) malnutrition should be dealt with before patients are admitted to hospital.

11 What does the writer say about ERAS protocols?

(A) They may be associated with a higher risk of infection.

(B) Their effectiveness has been demonstrated by his own experience.

(C) Their aim is different from that of preoperative protocols.

(D) They have been tested primarily on gastrointestinal patients.

12 In the fifth paragraph, the writer points out that

(A) reducing noise levels would be good for staff as well as patients.

(B) hospitals already have the information they need to improve patients' sleep.

(C) some of the measures designed to protect patients actually make them more ill.

(D) lack of action on the part of hospitals has led to patients finding ways to reduce noise disruption.

13 The '**default setting**' referred to in the fifth paragraph is

(A) writing down the results of regular checks on patients.

(B) writing down how often a patient should be checked.

(C) checking patients more often than every four hours.

(D) checking patients at four-hour intervals.

14 What does the writer propose in the final paragraph?

(A) surveying patients about how poor nutrition and sleep have affected them

(B) using medical journals to highlight the link between basic needs and treatment outcomes

(C) redesigning hospital buildings so they meet patients' needs more effectively

(D) gathering more evidence of the importance of needs such as sleep and nutrition

Text 2: Heading, concussion and dementia: how medicine is changing football forever

Football, particularly the act of heading, has been linked to damage to players' brains since 2014, when a coroner attributed England Striker Jeff Astle's death to **'industrial disease'** (one of the standard short form conclusions used by coroners) from repeated heading. Studies found that Astle's brain showed signs of chronic traumatic encephalopathy (CTE), a neurodegenerative disease commonly seen in boxers. Since then, other studies have investigated the connection with football, and 'a growing scientific consensus' exists that heading increases the risk of dementia, says Gill Livingston, a professor of psychiatry of older people.

Risk factors for dementia include traumatic brain injury, CTE, alcohol misuse, diet, air pollution, lack of education and genetics. The decision to include CTE was steered by the FIELD study (Football's InfluencE on Lifelong health and Dementia risk), which compared health records for 7,676 male, ex-professional football players who mostly played between 1950 and 1980 with 23,028 people from the general population of the same age, sex, and socio-demographic profile. Unsurprisingly, it found that football was beneficial to health. The footballers lived longer and were less likely to die of heart disease or lung cancer. But they were also 3.5 times more likely to die of dementia. The finding sparked concern and the establishment of new commissions, studies, regulations, and difficult and unresolved discussions over the sport's future.

The footballers' lifestyle – they were notorious in their era for drinking and smoking – may have played a role, says Peter Passmore, who studies cognitive disorders and dementia. The study looked at a broad range of disparate neurodegenerative disorders, including dementia, motor neuron disease, and Parkinson's. Most identified causes of dementia are associations rather than proven risk factors, and it is therefore difficult to establish the role football plays. 'There are tonnes of associations with dementia. It's nearly impossible to determine cause and effect,' says Passmore.

In order to pinpoint the cause of the increased risk of neurodegenerative disorders, the footballers' playing positions were factored in. Outfield players would be expected to have a higher risk as they head the ball more, but the difference was remarkable, according to Doug Smith, professor of neurosurgery. Defenders, who head the ball most, were five times more likely to develop dementia than the general population. For midfielders it was 4.59, for forwards (strikers) 2.79 and for goalkeepers, who almost never head the ball, 1.83. For all players, the longer their football career, the higher their chance of developing a neurodegenerative disease. 'I hadn't expected such clear results,' says Smith. 'On the other hand, I'm not surprised that at least for a certain number of individuals, having multiple, serious head impacts has a bad effect.'

Increasingly, evidence suggests that sub-concussive blows could have a more subtle but cumulative effect than concussion. 'Anybody who really studies this field is convinced that there's a link [between dementia and heading],' Smith says. His theory is that when players clash heads, the rapid acceleration damages axons in the brain. How much force is required and exactly how it damages the brain is unknown. Is it a single head acceleration that leads to either short-term or long-term neurodegeneration, or the density of a lot of little hits? **'The jury's still out'** says Arbogast.

In 2018, the US National Football League (NFL) banned certain tackles and moves, resulting in a reduction in collision speeds. The rule amendments were prompted by studies showing collisions between players were causing concussion and increased risk of brain damage. The modifications had little effect on the way the game is played, says Arbogast, who, as a consultant for the NFL Players Association, identified the cause of concussion in the game. But concussion dropped

35% on the previous season, to the lowest rate ever recorded. Improved equipment is also helping and discussion is ongoing over whether to prohibit tackles at younger ages.

The question is whether the time has come for the European version of football to consider similar changes, with heading the most obvious target. Arbogast and Smith say more research should be carried out, with the results informing adaptations in the game in order to minimise risk. That could mean improved equipment, rule changes, or better training on the signs and symptoms of concussion. Consultants should be brought in to work closely with football as they do in the NFL. Smith believes it is too early to remove heading from the sport, and is concerned that people are being scared away. 'I get emails from young footballers who are concerned, but the game has enormous health benefits,' says Smith. 'It would be sad if they dropped the game altogether.' Arbogast points out that footballers have better cardiovascular health, are less likely to be overweight, and gain leadership, soft skills, and social bonds. But it does seem the time has come to ask tough questions and start exploring the answers: can the game live without heading, particularly if it means players can live on?

Text 2: Questions 15–22

15 What do we learn about Jeff Astle?

(A) His brain injuries resembled those typically suffered by boxers.

(B) His death led to more research into the link between football and dementia.

(C) The cause of death originally given for him was changed on further investigation.

(D) He was the first footballer to claim that his dementia was caused by heading a ball.

16 What is suggested about the writer's attitude towards the phrase **industrial disease**?

(A) He assumes it is a carefully considered explanation.

(B) He believes it shows the coroner wasn't thorough enough.

(C) He doesn't feel it is completely appropriate in this case.

(D) He thinks it effectively highlights the seriousness of the findings.

17 According to the writer, the FIELD study

(A) had its results challenged by later research.

(B) didn't include data from a wide enough range of people.

(C) didn't reveal any new findings about football and dementia.

(D) has raised questions about the action football authorities need to take.

18 What is explained in the third paragraph?

(A) what the difference is between a risk factor and an association

(B) why it's hard to be sure that football increases the risk of dementia

(C) which other neurodegenerative disorders have been linked to football

(D) how the typical lifestyle of a footballer is more relevant to dementia than the game itself

19 What was Doug Smith's reaction to the research?

(A) He was shocked by how conclusive its findings were.

(B) He was pleased that it supported his own theory.

(C) He was unconvinced by the methodology used.

(D) He was puzzled by some of the data gathered.

20 The phrase **The jury's still out** in the fifth paragraph suggests that questions remain regarding

(A) how new evidence can be gathered.

(B) what type of impact leads to dementia.

(C) how to explain findings to non-scientists.

(D) whether other experts will accept Smith's theory.

21 What do we learn about the changes that the NFL have made?

(A) Their impact on play has been minimal.

(B) They were requested by players themselves.

(C) They will soon become obligatory for younger players.

(D) Their introduction has led to the redesigning of equipment.

22 According to the final paragraph, both Arbogast and Smith

(A) believe it's necessary to ban heading in football.

(B) wish to stress the advantages of playing football.

(C) encourage young players to find ways to play football safely.

(D) would value the opinions of the consultants used by the NFL.

TIME ALLOWED: **READING TIME:**   **5 MINUTES**

                        WRITING TIME: **40 MINUTES**

Read the case notes and complete the writing task which follows.

Notes:

Assume that today's date is 23 December 2016.

You are a family doctor treating a 33-year-old female patient who has been registered at your practice since childhood.

PATIENT DETAILS:

Name:	Lucy Smith (Ms)
DOB:	19 February 1983 (33 y.o.)
Address:	49 Whitehall Rd, Newtown

Social background: Primary school principal (busy, stressful job, long hours)

                               Married, (husband 39 y.o., Sales Director)

                               1 child (7 y.o.)

                               Enjoys live music concerts

                               Alcohol: approx.10 units/wk (mainly wine)

                               Non smoker

Allergies: Contact dermatitis (trigger = fragrance in soap, treatment = topical steroids)

Family History: Unremarkable

Past medical history: Astigmatism (wears glasses)

                               Greenstick fracture L ulna shaft (11 y.o.)

Treatment record:

10 Sept 2016:   Over-the-counter pregnancy test positive

                               Ordered blood test to confirm, CBC & BMP (basic metabolic panel)

                               Height: 165cm, Weight: 80kg, BMI: 29.4 (overweight)

                               Discussion:

                               Diet: convenience foods, e.g., ready-made meals (dislikes fresh veg), full-sugar soft drinks (dislikes sugar-free equivalents)

                               Weight loss attempts (last 5 yrs): various diets, low-calorie to low-protein = all unsuccessful

20 Sept 2016:   Blood test confirmed pregnancy, other results in normal range

                               BP 120/80 (normal)

                               Ultrasound referral

20 Oct 2016:	Ultrasound: 2nd trimester – healthy baby

22 Nov 2016:	Reported ↑frequent urination & ↑thirst (no change in diet, exercise level, medication, stress level or lifestyle)
	OGTT (Oral Glucose Tolerance Test) ordered

3 Dec 2016:	OGTT: gestational diabetes diag.
	Advice: healthy eating habits (pamphlets & fact sheets given), diet plan to limit weight gain during pregnancy
	Continuous glucose monitoring (CGM) device given to pt (= sensor under skin, displays levels on smartphone w alarm if too high)
	BP 130/80
	Repeat OGTT in 3 wks

23 Dec 2016:	OGTT results: blood glucose = 160 mg/dL (above normal levels)
	Discussion:
	Diet - no changes, reasons given = lack of time, busy w work, can't cook for husband/child/herself separately
	Explained insulin injections needed if no dietary changes made, pt reluctant:
	'I hate injections'
	Recommend dietitian referral, pt agrees

Plan:	Refer to dietitian for further support

Writing Task:

Using the information in the case notes, write a letter of referral to Ms Chakrabati, dietitian, outlining the patient's relevant medical background and requesting dietary management and support. Address the letter to Ms Meghna Chakrabati, Dietitian, Newtown Hospital, 123 High Street, Newtown.

In your answer:
- **Expand the relevant notes into complete sentences**
- **Do not use note form**
- **Use letter format**

The body of the letter should be approximately 180–200 words.

Part A

In this part of the test, you'll hear two different extracts. In each extract, a health professional is talking to a patient.

For **questions 1–24**, complete the notes with information you hear.

Now, look at the notes for extract one.

Extract 1: Questions 1–12

You hear an ophthalmologist talking to a patient called Myra Sudborne. For **questions 1–12**, complete the notes with a word or short phrase that you hear.

You now have thirty seconds to look at the notes.

Patient:	Myra Sudborrne

Onset of condition:
- noticed **(1)** _____ in peripheral vision
- diagnosis of glaucoma
- prescribed eye drops (no improvement)
  - led to frequent headaches and episodes of **(2)** _____
- now seeing a **(3)** _____ around lights
- believes her vision is deteriorating

Family history:
- mother diagnosed with both glaucoma and **(4)** _____
  - eventually total loss of vision
- maternal aunt had cataract surgery
- father wore **(5)** _____ for poor eyesight

Medical history:
- **(6)** _____ (thirty years ago)
- COPD – heavy smoker until recently (since teens)
- recent **(7)** _____ infection (hospital admission)
- hearing aids – rarely wears them
- frequent **(8)** _____ (last twelve months)

Current Medication:
- three courses of antibiotics (last six months)
- uses her **(9)** _____ regularly
- theophylline
- recently received **(10)** _____ vaccine

Patient concerns: eyesight problems affecting ability to cope at home –
- no longer able to **(11)** _____
- feels generally vulnerable
- now considering **(12)** _____ (admits to feeling reluctant)

Extract 2: Questions 13–24

You hear a neurologist talking to a patient called Justin Blake. For questions 13–24, complete the notes with a word or short phrase that you hear.

You now have thirty seconds to look at the notes.

Patient: Justin Blake

Current symptoms:

- diagnosis of Parkinson's Disease (three years ago)

- speech has become noticeably **(13)** _____

- experiencing insomnia and feels constantly cold

- sensation of **(14)** _____ (right side of body)

- occasional difficulties with **(15)** _____

Impact on everyday life:

- mentions **(16)** _____ as an activity he can no longer do

- some absences from work – attributed to **(17)** _____

- hasn't experienced **(18)** _____ to date

- maintains an active social life

- has developed a **(19)** _____ (makes him self-conscious)

Medication:

- taking carbidopa-levodopa – no issues

- **(20)** _____ at bedtime (commenced recently)

- Ibuprofen for general discomfort

- requests something to treat **(21)** _____

Lifestyle factors:

- not prepared to reduce **(22)** _____

- has recently stopped **(23)** _____

- resumed smoking (two months ago)

- requests a **(24)** _____ referral

Part B

In this part of the test, you'll hear six different extracts. In each extract, you'll hear people talking in a different healthcare setting.

For **questions 25–30**, choose the answer (**A**, **B** or **C**) which fits best according to what you hear. You'll have time to read each question before you listen. Complete your answers as you listen.

Now look at question 25.

 Fill the circle in completely. Example:

25 You hear a senior paediatric nurse briefing a colleague about a patient on their ward.

What does the colleague agree to do?

(A) request a review of the patient's medication

(B) show the patient how to self-administer medication

(C) reassure the patient's family about aspects of his care plan

26 You hear a hospital doctor talking to a patient who's just given birth.

What is she asking him to do?

(A) check that her sutures are intact

(B) agree for her to be discharged

(C) prescribe some medication

27 You hear a senior nurse in a care home for the elderly briefing a new team member.

What is she explaining about mealtimes?

- (A) what to do if a patient seems to need special equipment
- (B) how to identify those patients who may need assistance
- (C) why the needs of certain patient groups are prioritised

28 You hear an oncologist talking to a hospital pharmacist about a patient's medication.
The pharmacist is going to find out whether

- (A) an alternative to the medication is available.
- (B) it's still possible to administer the medication.
- (C) the medication is available in another formulation.

29 You hear a primary-care doctor leaving a voicemail message for a community nurse.

What is the priority for the patient?

- (A) collecting a sample for further investigations
- (B) providing therapy for a pre-existing condition
- (C) changing the dressings on a long-standing wound

30 You hear part of a briefing meeting for nursing staff at a primary-care practice.

What is the speaker doing?

- (A) explaining why nasal sprays are often thought ineffective
- (B) discouraging discussion of nasal sprays with patient's parents
- (C) reminding them why certain nasal sprays shouldn't be recommended

Part C

In this part of the test, you'll hear two different extracts. In each extract, you'll hear health professionals talking about aspects of their work.

For **questions 31–42**, choose the answer (**A, B** or **C**) which fits best according to what you hear. Complete your answers as you listen.

Now look at extract one.

 Fill the circle in completely. Example:

Extract 1: Questions 31–36

You hear an oncologist called Dr Hannah Owen giving a presentation about a new treatment method called a chemotherapy backpack.

You now have 90 seconds to read **questions 31–36**.

31   Dr Owen suggests the main advantage of the backpack for patients is that it

   (A)   reduces the wider impact of treatment.

   (B)   benefits those who are most vulnerable.

   (C)   means they can control their own medication.

32   Dr Owen explains that to qualify for a backpack, patients need to

   (A)   understand exactly how the equipment works.

   (B)   distinguish between different warning signals.

   (C)   have full-time support in place at home.

33   Patient feedback on the backpack has suggested that it

   (A)   allows most patients to become more active.

   (B)   motivates patients to maintain their independence.

   (C)   helps patients to deal with side effects of their treatment.

34 Dr Owen mentions a patient called Kieran to show how using a backpack can

(A) take the pressure off other family members.

(B) help develop the patients' understanding of the illness.

(C) convince employers to allow patients to continue working.

35 For the patient called Jessica, the main advantage of having a chemotherapy backpack was that

(A) she could limit the time she spent away from home.

(B) she felt well enough to do some domestic chores.

(C) she was able to avoid relying on childcare.

36 Dr Owen hopes that in the future, the backpack will

(A) be used for a wider range of conditions.

(B) gain greater popularity amongst patients.

(C) become more cost effective for hospitals.

Now look at extract two.

Extract 2: Questions 37–42

You hear an interview with a nurse called Adam Bojani, who's developed a hand hygiene resource pack aimed at children.

You now have 90 seconds to read questions **37–42**.

37 What point does Adam make about children in relation to hand hygiene and the spread of disease?

   (A) They're unaware how the two things are related.

   (B) They aren't motivated to follow routines that protect others.

   (C) They can't be expected to adopt new habits without support.

38 Adam team decided to develop their resource pack for children because they

   (A) had access to some interesting new technology.

   (B) felt existing materials were rather old fashioned.

   (C) realised the issue wasn't being adequately addressed.

39 What aspect of the project's implementation does Adam see as particularly worthwhile?

   (A) its potential impact in highly vulnerable communities

   (B) how well non-specialised staff have delivered it

   (C) the accessibility of the material across cultures

40 Adam feels the involvement of nurses in the project is important because they

(A) have experience in patient education initiatives.

(B) will be needed to help establish it in hospitals.

(C) often work in a range of community settings.

41 The effectiveness of the resource pack was assessed by

(A) asking children themselves to give feedback.

(B) analysing how well children followed selected routines.

(C) monitoring how carefully children applied what they'd learned.

42 Initial findings indicate that the project's impact on infection rates

(A) is difficult to measure in the short term.

(B) has extended beyond the immediate participants.

(C) could have an influence on wider policy making in the future.

OET SAMPLE TEST

ROLEPLAYER CARD NO. 1	MEDICINE

SETTING   Doctor's Clinic

PATIENT   You are 42 years old and have been experiencing fatigue for the last three months. The doctor has just finished examining you.

TASK
- When asked, say you wake up hourly most nights. You usually go to sleep at midnight after watching TV. You get up at 8:00am. You don't nap during the day and your spouse hasn't reported that you snore.

- When asked, say you eat plenty of red meat, fruit and vegetables, but you don't have the energy to do any exercise. You watch TV in bed when you get home from work and drink coffee to stay awake. You don't have much stress.

- Say the doctor must be able to tell you now what he/she thinks is wrong with you.

- Say you'll follow the doctor's advice. Ask if there's anything else you can do.

- Say you are ready to have the blood test, and you'll make the follow-up appointment.

© Cambridge Boxhill Language Assessment (2022)   SAMPLE TEST

OET SAMPLE TEST

CANDIDATE CARD NO. 1	MEDICINE

SETTING   Doctor's Clinic

DOCTOR   This 42-year-old patient has suffered from fatigue for the last three months. You have just finished examining the patient and have found no abnormalities.

TASK
- Find out about patient's sleep (e.g., quality, duration, daytime naps, possible snoring, etc.).

- Explore lifestyle factors (e.g., diet, exercise, screen time, caffeine-intake, stress, etc.).

- Recommend further investigation (e.g., blood test: complete blood count, thyroid function test, serum vitamin D, etc.).

- Reassure patient about fatigue (e.g., typically combination lifestyle/social/psychological cause, often no underlying medical condition, etc.). Advise on improving sleep hygiene (e.g., no electronics in bedroom, no screens/caffeine before sleeping, get up if not asleep within 20 minutes, etc.).

- Recommend lifestyle modifications (e.g., increased physical activity, relaxation techniques before bed, etc.). Outline next steps (e.g., blood test, follow-up appointment in three days for results, etc.).

© Cambridge Boxhill Language Assessment (2022)   SAMPLE TEST

ROLEPLAYER CARD NO. 2   MEDICINE

SETTING	Doctor's Clinic
PATIENT	You are 21 years old and you have a painful lump on your wrist. The doctor has just finished examining your wrist.
TASK	• When asked, say you first noticed the lump while playing tennis about two months ago. It's grown bigger since then. It hurts to move your wrist.
	• When asked, say you work in a restaurant. You carry heavy plates and do lots of lifting and cleaning.
	• Say your father told you to hit the lump with a heavy book to push it back in. You've been thinking of trying that.
	• When asked, say you'd like to have the lump removed using the needle.
	• Say you'll use a wrist brace and will come back next week for the procedure.

© Cambridge Boxhill Language Assessment (2022)   SAMPLE TEST

CANDIDATE CARD NO. 2   MEDICINE

SETTING	Doctor's Clinic
DOCTOR	This 21-year-old patient has a painful lump on his/her wrist. You have just finished examining the wrist. You diagnose a ganglion cyst.
TASK	• Find out more details about lump on patient's wrist (e.g., onset, changes, pain, etc.).
	• Explore further relevant details about patient (e.g., work, use of wrist/hand, etc.).
	• Give diagnosis of ganglion cyst (e.g., benign fluid-filled sac, small tear in tendon membrane allowing contents to protrude, possibly caused by trauma to wrist, often self-limiting etc.). Recommend pain management (e.g., brace/splint immobilisation, paracetamol if required, etc.).
	• Advise against self-treatment of cyst (e.g., further damage to surrounding area, likelihood of recurrence, etc.). Explain options for cyst removal (e.g., needle aspiration, surgery as final option, etc.). Establish patient's preference for treatment of cyst.
	• Outline next steps (e.g., appointment for aspiration next week, wrist brace beneficial before/after procedure, etc.).

© Cambridge Boxhill Language Assessment (2022)   SAMPLE TEST

Pyelonephritis: Texts

Text A

Acute pyelonephritis is an infection within the renal pelvis and the renal parenchyma – the functioning part of the kidney responsible for filtering blood and producing urine. It is most often caused by ascending infection from the bladder but haematogenous spread can also occur.

- The usual organisms involved are the same as for lower urinary tract infection (UTI) – e.g. E. coli.
- Unusual organisms are occasionally seen – e.g. mycobacteria, yeasts and fungi and opportunistic pathogens such as *Corynebacterium urealyticum.*

- Repeated attacks can lead to chronic pyelonephritis, which involves destruction and scarring of renal tissue.

Acute pyelonephritis can occur at any age. Around 1% of boys and 3% of girls will have had acute pyelonephritis by the age of 7. Incidence is highest in women aged 15–29, followed by infants and older people. It is relatively uncommon in men. In neonates it is more common in boys and tends to be associated with abnormalities of the renal tract. Over the age of 65 the incidence in men rises to match that of women.

Text B

Investigations

Urinalysis	• Urine is often cloudy with an offensive smell • Dipstick Avenir LT Std may be positive for blood, protein, leukocyte esterase and nitrite. • Midstream urine specimen must be sent for microscopy and culture. • Catheter specimen will be acceptable if a catheter is in situ (collection bag or pad may be used when a sample is not obtainable by superior means). • Microscopy of urine specimen shows pyuria.
Inflammatory markers	C-reactive protein (CRP), erythrocyte sedimentation rate (ESR), and plasma viscosity may be raised.
Blood cultures	Positive in approximately 15–30% of cases.
Ultrasonography	Normally recommended for men and children. Is usually the first-line investigation – mandatory in patients with recurrent pyelonephritis – may help to identify obstruction or stones.
CECT scan	The best investigation in adults where diagnosis is in doubt, improvement does not occur after 72 hours of treatment, or deterioration occurs.
MRI	Useful in detecting scarring. May require sedation in children. In adults, it is increasingly used where renal infection and urinary obstruction are suspected. Preferred in pregnant women.

Text C

Presentation

Onset is usually rapid with symptoms appearing over a day or two. There is unilateral or bilateral loin pain, suprapubic pain or back pain. Fever is variable but can be high enough to produce rigors. Malaise, nausea, vomiting, anorexia and occasionally diarrhoea occur. There may or may not be accompanying lower urinary tract symptoms with frequency, burning, tingling, or stinging sensations (dysuria), blood in the stream, or hesitancy. The patient looks ill and there is commonly pain on firm palpation of one or both kidneys and moderate suprapubic tenderness without guarding.

Presentation in children, especially when young, can be much less specific and urine culture should be a routine investigation in pyrexial and unwell infants.

Common differential diagnoses may include:

- Cystitis.
- Ectopic pregnancy.
- Ovarian torsion.
- Ruptured ovarian cyst.

- Rib fracture.
- STDs.
- Renal stone.
- Benign prostatic hyperplasia.

Text D

Management

Support: rest, adequate fluid intake and analgesia are important.

Hospital admission: indications for admission include:

- Severe vomiting, pain or debility.
- Signs of sepsis (eg, tachycardia, hypotension).
- Urinary tract obstruction.
- No response to treatment > 24 hours.
- Pregnancy

- Dehydration
- Non-concordance with treatment.
- Inadequate access to follow-up.
- Relapse when antibiotics are stopped.

All babies aged under 3 months should be admitted.

Antibiotics:

Adults	Dose	Duration	Notes
Ciprofloxacin	500 mg 2x daily	7 days	
(or) Co-amoxiclav	500/125 mg 3x daily		
Trimethoprim	200 mg 2x daily	14 days	May be used if culture confirms effectiveness
Children			
Co-amoxiclav	**Child < 5 years** 0.25 mL/kilogram 3x daily		By mouth using oral suspension 125/31 Dose doubled in severe infection.
	Child 6–11 years 0.15 mL/kilogram 3x daily		By mouth using oral suspension 250/62 Dose doubled in severe infection.
	Child 12–15 years 250/125 mg 3x daily **Child 16 17 years** 500/125 mg 3x daily	7–10 days	By mouth using tablets

Part A

TIME: 15 minutes

- Look at the four texts, **A–D**, in the separate **Text Booklet** that precedes the questions.

- For each question, **1–20**, look through the texts, **A–D**, to find the relevant information.

- Write your answers on the spaces provided in this **Question Paper**.

- Answer all the questions within the 15-minute time limit.

- Your answers should **only** be taken from texts **A–D** and must be correctly spelt.

Pyelonephritis: Questions

Questions 1–7

For each question, **1–7**, decide which text (**A**, **B**, **C** or **D**) the information comes from. You may use any letter more than once.

In which text can you find information about

    1   the advantages of different types of examinations for pyelonephritis?   _____

    2   symptoms that may indicate a patient with pyelonephritis needs in-patient care?   _____

    3   conditions for which pyelonephritis may be mistaken?   _____

    4   where in the kidneys pyelonephritis occurs?   _____

    5   a problem with diagnosing pyelonephritis in younger patients?   _____

    6   the health consequences of recurrent pyelonephritis in an individual?   _____

    7   the length of time that pyelonephritis medications need to be taken for?   _____

Questions 8–13

Answer each of the questions, **8–13**, with a word or short phrase from one of the texts. Each answer may include words, numbers or both.

    8   In what form is co-amoxiclav administered to children over 12 years old?

    _____

    9   What complication of pyelonephritis is suggested by hypotension?

    _____

10 What is the recommended single dose per kilogram of 250/62 co-amoxiclav for a 9-year-old child?

_____

11 What effect of fever may be observed in patients presenting with pyelonephritis?

_____

12 What type of imaging test is suggested initially for male patients with suspected pyelonephritis?

_____

13 Which age group of women is most at risk from pyelonephritis?

_____

Questions 14–20

Complete each of the sentences, **14–20**, with a word or short phrase from one of the texts. Each answer may include words, numbers or both.

14 If _____ of either kidney causes pain, this may indicate pyelonephritis.

15 _E. coli_ can be a common factor in both _____ and pyelonephritis.

16 Acute Pyelonephritis usually results from an infection which began in the patient's

_____

17 The presence of blood in a patient's urine can be confirmed if _____ is positive.

18 A _____ should be performed to resolve an uncertain pyelonephritis diagnosis in an adult.

19 Urine samples obtained from a _____ are preferred to samples from a collection bag.

20 If testing indicates it is suitable, _____ may be used to treat pyelonephritis in adults.

Part B

In this part of the test, there are six short extracts relating to the work of health professionals.

For **questions 1–6**, choose the answer (**A**, **B** or **C**) which you think fits best according to the text.

Fill the circle in completely. Example:

---

1   The purpose of this guideline on the use of anaesthetic gas is to

   (A)   emphasise the importance of patient safety during its administration.

   (B)   identify those patients who are most at risk after it has been used during a procedure.

   (C)   clarify the criteria for deciding whether patients who have received it can perform certain tasks.

Safe use of Entonox gas for short term pain relief

Patient Information

All patients receiving Entonox must be given verbal and written information (via patient information leaflet LN 1215, available on the hospital intranet) regarding the drug. When Entonox is used as a sole analgesic/sedative agent, driving and use of complex machinery is not recommended until:

- at least 30 minutes has elapsed after the administration of Entonox has ceased
- the healthcare professional has assessed that the patient has returned to normal mental status i.e. orientated to time and place
- the patient feels that they are competent to drive or use machinery after the relevant procedure is completed. i.e there is no residual drowsiness or light headedness.

Additional care is needed when Entonox is administered to a patient who has been given associated medication.

---

2   The extract from the policy on adult patients who go missing emphasises the importance of

   (A)   establishing the likelihood of this as soon as possible.

   (B)   enabling staff to visually identify patients at most risk of this.

   (C)   working with relatives in order to locate patients who have done this.

Adult Missing Patient Policy

An assessment on admission may determine whether the patient has confusion, memory problems, depression and/or is a risk to themselves; these are all indicators of an increased risk of them going missing from hospital. This assessment should include any previous history and/or patterns of going missing and should be completed in collaboration with the patient, and/or with input from family or a designated contact. Patients whose mental health status may change rapidly due to their medical condition may require repeated risk assessments over the day. Medical and nursing staff must undertake this jointly and the outcome must be recorded in the patient's clinical record. In clinical areas, all in-patients must wear a wristband that includes forename, surname, date of birth, id number and gender. For patients identified as 'high risk', it is good practice to ensure that their wristbands also include details of their current care location.

3　The email about Just in Case Boxes includes information on

   (A)　the rationale for providing them.

   (B)　a change in policy regarding them.

   (C)　some concerns raised about them.

To:	Staff working off-site
From:	Hospital board
Subject:	Just in Case Boxes

Like many areas nationally, we are now developing a system of Just in Case Boxes to support anticipatory prescribing and access to palliative care medication for patients with common symptoms in the end-of-life phase e.g. pain, agitation, breathlessness, and nausea. Adequate quantities of the appropriate medicines will be prescribed for the patient and stored in an identifiable container, the 'Just in Case Box', in the patient's home. Carers and patients need to be reassured that the prescribed medicines have been prescribed 'just in case', and may not be needed. Patients and carers will be provided with a contact phone number to ensure timely access to symptom assessment and management.

4　The guideline on summoning clinical assistance stresses the importance of

   (A)　contacting the medical staff currently treating the patient.

   (B)　following a set procedure in order to obtain assistance.

   (C)　providing immediate first aid until help arrives.

Summoning clinical assistance

If someone is found collapsed, not breathing normally or requires urgent medical assistance, dial 2222 straightaway and ask for the Cardiac Arrest Team. This may involve leaving the person alone.

* Inform the switchboard whether the person is an adult or a child.
* On return to the person, commence emergency life support if required.

The Cardiac Arrest team leader will be responsible for further assessment of the patient in liaison with other relevant specialties and decide on the most appropriate area to transfer the patient for further assessment or care.

If Emergency Department (ED) advice is then required, call the ED on 6699. If the ambulance service is required, provide ambulance control staff with clear and concise clinical information as requested along with directions to the site of the incident. Avoid using abbreviations.

5 The purpose of the extract from the policy on seasonal influenza management is to

  Ⓐ explain the procedure for establishing isolation facilities.

  Ⓑ identify the staff responsible for moving patients into isolation.

  Ⓒ outline the procedures for the care of patients in isolation.

Seasonal influenza management policy

Isolation

Patients with suspected flu will be admitted to a single room. Patients with confirmed flu will remain isolated in a single room or cohort bay for the duration of their infectious period, or until discharged. If a patient requires ventilatory support, a negative pressure room in the ICU should be used. In such cases, a discussion between a respiratory physician and site management must happen. If it becomes necessary, sufficient single rooms or cohort areas will be designated for patients with confirmed and suspected flu by the hospital management. Isolation patients may undergo investigations in other departments, provided the relevant department has received advance notification. While outside isolation, the patient should wear a surgical face mask. The area and any equipment that the patient has been in contact with should be appropriately decontaminated on completion of the investigation.

---

6 The extract from a pulse oximeter manual includes a reminder that the device

  Ⓐ may stop working without warning in some circumstances.

  Ⓑ may still be used when its internal power supply is unavailable.

  Ⓒ may be irreparably damaged if it is left to recharge for too long.

Pulse Oximeter Manual
Recharging the battery

When new and charged to full capacity, the oximeter's internal battery provides at least 5½ hours of continuous operation, at normal temperatures. A LOW BATTERY message appears when 5 to 15 minutes of battery operation remain. When the alarm message CONNECT UNIT TO LINE POWER appears during operation on battery power, an audible alarm sounds and the oximeter automatically shuts off in approximately 10 seconds.

Important: To prevent permanent loss of capacity, recharge a discharged battery within eight hours after the LOW BATTERY message is displayed. To recharge, plug the oximeter into the AC power supply (approximately 8 hours for 100% capacity). Note that the oximeter remains operational while recharging the battery. The battery will not overcharge. Batteries stored for extended periods of time should be recharged every six months to maintain their charging capacity.

In this part of the test, there are two texts about different aspects of healthcare. For questions **7–22**, choose the answer (**A**, **B**, **C** or **D**) which you think fits best according to the text.

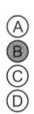

Fill the circle in completely. Example:

Text 1: Can 'lifestyle medicine' help treat chronic pain?

Like 2.2 million Australians, Anu Kulkarni has osteoarthritis. Her knee and foot joints are painfully inflamed. Having spent almost three decades dealing with chronic pain, Anu says, 'medication is what keeps me going. If I wasn't to take the painkillers, I might be struggling to walk.' She also experiences depression and anxiety, and for a two-year period, was unable to leave home. Now, she and husband Narendra have signed up for an eight-week experiment to make some lifestyle changes with the help of Dr Preeya Alexander.

Chronic pain, such as that experienced by patients with osteoarthritis, is typically defined by its duration — anything over three months is usually considered chronic. It's incredibly complex but according to neuroscientist Dr Tasha Stanton, if we can change how we understand pain and what contributes to it, we can reduce our experience of it. 'We're feeling pain because our brain is determining whether or not we need to be protected,' Dr Stanton says. But she thinks that in people with chronic pain, this is working too well.

For someone with osteoarthritis, pain is characterised by body-wide, low-level inflammation that can actually change the function of many of the body's systems such as the brain and the gut. Dr Stanton claims such changes influence the sensitivity of our pain systems. While all this means there are numerous different contributors to chronic pain, it also means there are numerous treatment targets. Interventions, such as alterations to diet are, she thinks, 'surprisingly more effective than most people think. They might not seem like much, but when you add them together … that can be an enormous contribution.'

Depression and anxiety can also have a significant impact on how someone experiences chronic pain. 'There are a lot of people who will say, "I notice when I'm feeling really stressed, when I'm feeling really anxious, when my mood is really, really low, that my pain is worse,"' Dr Stanton says. When someone with chronic pain, like Anu, also experiences anxiety, 'it blocks our natural drug cabinet in the brain,' she says. But the good news is that because chronic pain management is multifaceted, she says **this** can be controlled to some extent — the brain isn't fixed, but can be reoriented. Dr Preeya Alexander appears to concur. She thinks that something everyone can do in these increasingly hectic times is to make time to be quiet and calm. She goes on to say that 'people who suffer with anxiety show increased activity in the amygdala — a part of the brain that regulates the fear response. Practising mindfulness meditation can dampen that activity and increase a person's ability to regulate their emotions.'

Anu says that during her two years at home, she experienced the greatest pain she's ever known. This period was also marked by weight gain – something she's struggled with ever since. Her efforts led her into a damaging pattern of skipping meals and eating protein supplements when hungry. 'I have been eating [them] because they say banana is fattening,' Anu says. Dr Alexander brings in nutritionist Simran Grover to challenge this assumption. Ms Grover suggests simple changes to Anu's diet, such as swapping protein supplements for fruit. While we often think of weight gain putting pressure on our joints, Dr Stanton says, we're starting to learn more about its contribution to inflammation as a whole. This may explain why, for instance, people can feel pain in joints they don't bear weight on.

Exercise is another key area for managing chronic pain. But Dr Stanton says fear is often a problem because in such cases, the pain system tends to be over-protective. 'What that means is that when you're starting to [exercise] and you do feel pain, you're nowhere near the level that it would take to damage tissue or to further injure yourself,' she says. 'You're doing activity at a level that actually you can be sore but you're safe, and that understanding is really important, because when we have increases in activity over time, there are positive adaptations in our pain system.' The key to exercising well for someone with chronic pain is gradual increases over time.

For Anu, the real test of her work with Dr Alexander came when they met at the pool on the final day. After going through some of her mindfulness meditation techniques before they entered the water together, Anu began to float and the look on her face **said it all**. 'Being able to swim again, it's freedom.' While Anu is still on pain medication at the end of the experiment, she continues to practise mindfulness and has drastically cut her protein consumption. 'It's small steps … but we knew from the beginning, because I'm suffering from chronic pain, it's not just going to go away like that,' she says.

Text 1: Questions 7–14

7   What is the writer doing in the first paragraph?

   (A)   detailing the typical progress of osteoarthritis in a patient

   (B)   illustrating the value of pain medication to patients with osteoarthritis

   (C)   exemplifying the personal impact of osteoarthritis on health and wellbeing

   (D)   explaining the background to a new treatment for patients with osteoarthritis

8   In the second paragraph, the writer refers to Dr Stanton in order

   (A)   to explain why chronic pain tends to worsen over time.

   (B)   to identify the ultimate cause of chronic pain in an individual.

   (C)   to demonstrate that chronic pain is a physical rather than a mental issue.

   (D)   to show how new medical knowledge is changing the treatment of chronic pain.

9   What do we learn about lifestyle changes in the third paragraph?

   (A)   They tend to have a cumulative impact on pain.

   (B)   They have their greatest effect on the internal organs.

   (C)   They have to be carefully matched to particular causes of pain.

   (D)   They are rarely put into practice by those they would most benefit.

10 In the fourth paragraph, the word '**this**' refers to

(A) understanding the causes of anxiety.

(B) the nature of chronic pain.

(C) the way the brain works.

(D) the use of pain relief drugs.

11 In the fourth paragraph, the writer suggests Dr Stanton and Dr Alexander agree that

(A) the mental aspect of chronic pain is under-appreciated by most people.

(B) brain training should form a part of chronic pain management strategies.

(C) modern lifestyles are a major contributor to the widespread incidence of chronic pain.

(D) mindfulness can make people more willing to try new chronic pain management strategies.

12 What is the writer's main point in the fifth paragraph?

(A) People are generally ill-informed over the dangers of obesity.

(B) Being over-weight can have a wider impact than many people think.

(C) The impact of loneliness on people's eating habits is underestimated.

(D) Dietary products may have a negative impact on people with chronic pain.

13 In the sixth paragraph, what problem does Dr Stanton say might affect people with chronic pain who are taking exercise?

(A) Their own bodies may mislead them into giving up too early.

(B) The main obstacle they face is the psychological barrier of beginning.

(C) They sometimes fail to pay attention to important warning signs.

(D) There is a tendency for them to adopt over-ambitious schedules.

14 In the final paragraph, the expression '**said it all**' is used to express

(A) the amount of effort Anu has made to improve her condition.

(B) the value of the various relaxation techniques Anu has learned.

(C) the enjoyment Anu has derived from her time with Dr Alexander.

(D) the feeling of satisfaction Anu has with the results of her treatment.

Text 2: Predicting side effects of medication

A multi-institutional group of researchers has created an open-source machine learning tool that offers a new method for developing safer medicines by identifying potential adverse reactions – side effects – in new candidate medicines. One of the researchers, genetics expert Robert Ietswaart, says '**Machine learning is not a silver bullet** for drug discovery, but I do believe it can accelerate many different aspects in the difficult and long process of developing new medicines. Although it cannot predict all possible adverse effects, we hope that our work will help researchers spot potential trouble early on and develop safer drugs in the future.'

Adverse drug reactions, ranging from mild to fatal, may occur when taking a drug as prescribed, as well as through incorrect dosages, the interaction of multiple medicines or off-label use (taking a drug for something other than what it was approved for). In the USA alone, they cause 2 million hospitalizations each year and are a factor in up to 20 percent of hospitalizations, according to research. Researchers have applied many tactics to avoid or at least minimize these issues, but because a single drug often interacts with multiple proteins in the body – not always limited to the intended targets – identifying which of these was responsible can be hard if a drug does cause an adverse reaction. The same goes for predicting what, if any, side effects may happen.

The project was born three years ago when pharmacologist Laszlo Urban gave a presentation on some of the problems his team faces when assessing the safety of new drug candidates. A group of graduate and post-doctorate students then participated in a hackathon – an event in which people meet to carry out computer programming together. The aim was to apply their knowledge of data science and machine learning to the problem of creating an algorithm that could possibly predict adverse reactions to medication. Most of the time, such projects simply end up as learning exercises, but on this occasion, the interaction of scientists from different institutions actually generated a novel application published in a highly respected journal.

Following publication, the team began work on its machine learning algorithm and applied it to two large data sets: one from a pharmaceutical company concerning the proteins that each of 2,000 drugs interact with, and one from the U.S. Food and Drug Administration covering 600,000 physician reports of adverse drug reactions in patients. The computer algorithm was able to **connect the dots between them**. As it 'learned' from the data, the algorithm unearthed 221 associations which indicated which proteins may represent drug targets that currently contribute to particular side effects. Crucially, the information generated by the algorithm about how individual proteins, or the genes that make them, contribute to documented adverse reactions was statistically robust. Many of the results supported previous observations, such as the fact that certain drugs binding to the protein hERG can cause cardiac arrhythmias. Findings like this strengthened the researchers' confidence that the algorithm was performing well.

Some of the results generated by the algorithm were unexpected. For instance, the algorithm suggested that the protein PDE3 is associated with over 40 adverse drug reactions. Doctors and researchers have known for years that PDE3 inhibitors – common anti-clotting treatments for acute heart failure, stroke prevention and cardiogenic shock – can cause arrhythmias, low platelet counts and elevated levels of enzymes called transaminases, a possible indicator of liver damage. But it wasn't known that targeting PDE3 might expose patients to so many other adverse reactions, including some related to the muscles, bones, connective tissue, kidneys, urinary tract and ear.

Based on what it has already learned, as well as strengthened by as much new data as researchers can feed it, the algorithm appears to have raised the prospect that a potential new drug will prove safe for patients both before and after pharmaceutical companies bring it to market. This matters because it is something which could reduce the risks that study participants face during the first in-human clinical trials as well as minimizing risks for patients once a drug is approved for clinical use.

So, how accurate overall was the algorithm in terms of predicting the likelihood of a particular drug causing an adverse reaction? Until last year, the program had only learned from information on adverse reactions from a single 12-month period, six years earlier. The team then fed in figures from the next five years, some of which revealed side effects that hadn't been observed before from particular drugs. Sure enough, many of the algorithm's previously unproven predictions matched the recent real-world reports. 'What seemed like false-positive predictions proved not to be false at all when the new reports became available,' said Ietswaart. However, it is worth bearing in mind that although the researchers have strengthened the model as much as they could, it still assesses less than 1 percent of the human genome – the origin of the problematic proteins involved in adverse reactions. In the meantime, scientists can use, improve and build upon the model, which is posted for free online.

Text 2: Questions 15–22

15 When Robert Ietswaart says that says 'Machine learning is not a silver bullet' he is making the point that

    (A) it will only be a partial solution to the problems of developing new medication.

    (B) it is too early to be sure of its impact on the amount of research time required.

    (C) it is uncertain whether it will help to simplify medical research procedures.

    (D) it is unlikely to lead to the discovery of innovative new medications.

16 What is the writer's purpose in the second paragraph?

    (A) to describe some recent trends in the numbers of adverse drug reactions.

    (B) to summarise the difficulties involved in reducing adverse drug reactions.

    (C) to improve prescribing practices in order to reduce adverse drug reactions.

    (D) to outline various methods that have been used to reduce adverse drug reactions.

17 What does the writer say was unusual about the hackathon following Laszlo Urban's presentation?

    (A) the backgrounds of those that were involved

    (B) the speed with which it was carried out

    (C) the fact that it achieved a worthwhile result

    (D) the educational benefits for participants

18 The expression **connect the dots** refers to

    (A) confirming already suspected causes of adverse reactions.

    (B) finding potential new types of adverse reactions.

    (C) grouping harmful substances responsible for causing adverse reactions.

    (D) identifying links between results from two research projects into adverse reactions.

19 In the fourth paragraph, the writer says the team knew their algorithm was effective because

   (A) its findings were supported by information from government sources.

   (B) it agreed with findings from pharmaceutical manufacturers own research.

   (C) it confirmed a number of findings from existing research projects.

   (D) it passed a number of external analytical checks on its findings.

20 What does the writer say was unexpected about the findings regarding the protein PDE3?

   (A) the wide impact it has on the functioning of the body.

   (B) the implications for patients with reduced levels of it.

   (C) the severity of the side effects that it can cause in some drugs.

   (D) the number of health risks that can be associated with treatments related to it.

21 In the sixth paragraph, the writer makes the point that the computer algorithm

   (A) has already proved its ability to improve the safety of the subjects of research projects.

   (B) has had to be regularly updated with information in order to make progress.

   (C) is likely to change the way that patient studies are conducted in future.

   (D) would represent a major commercial breakthrough for drugs manufacturers.

22 What conclusion regarding the algorithm does the writer come to in the final paragraph?

   (A) The accuracy of its predictions has yet to be confirmed.

   (B) Its ability to predict side effects has exceeded all expectations.

   (C) It is still making its predictions using relatively limited data.

   (D) There is still work to be done to improve its reliability.

TIME ALLOWED: READING TIME: 5 MINUTES
WRITING TIME: 40 MINUTES

Read the case notes and complete the writing task which follows.

Notes:

Assume that today's date is 18 September 2018.
You are a family doctor examining an 80-year-old female who has been registered at your practice for 40 years.

PATIENT DETAILS:

Name:	Beryl Smith (Mrs)
DOB:	19 May 1938 (80 y.o.)
Address:	Rose Aged Care Home, 29 Rose Avenue, Newtown (moved there 2018)
Social background:	Retired librarian
	Widow (husband died 2016)
	3 daughters: Mary (lives abroad), Yana (died 2000, drowning), Susan (visits 1x/mth
	Interests: lawn bowls, playing cards, reading
	Note: support needed at external medical appts (Susan)
Family History:	Mother died 65 y.o. (blood clot)
	Father died 58 y.o. (alcoholic liver disease)
Past medical history:	2010 BCC (excision, no recurrence)
	2014 hypertension (controlled w ACE inhibitors)
	2016 L total hip replacement
	2017 ?dementia – initial stage ($\uparrow$forgetfulness, confusion)
	No known allergies
18 Sept 2018:	Pt accompanied by daughter
	<u>Presenting complaint</u>: ringing in ears (bilateral), mild headache, pruritus R ear
	<u>Objective:</u>
	Height: 153 cm, Weight: 55 kg, BMI: 23.5 kg/m^2 (normal)
	Bilateral otoscopy: normal tympanic membrane
	Rinne & Weber tests (normal)

Ear examination:

Definitive diagnosis:

        External configuration – R acute otitis externa (red, flaky, warm skin)

Provisional diagnosis:

        ?foreign bodies blocking R ear canal – ?cotton wool

        ?R otitis media (middle ear infection) – ?bacterial, ?fungal (request swab to confirm)

        ?bilateral hearing loss, ?tinnitus

Discussion:

Daughter – pt unable to hear questions/instructions if background noise (eg if radio on, in restaurants, when care home residents talk, etc.)

Pt – uses 'home remedies' (loud radio & cotton wool to block out ringing sound, honey for pruritus, moisturiser 2x/day for flaky skin)

Ceased social outings (cannot hear well outside)

Recommended: visual aids for use by care home staff (to communicate daily activities, instructions, etc)

Treatment: start antibiotic drops (potential otitis media to be confirmed by swab) & paracetamol 4x/day (headache)

Refer to audiologist for opinion & diagnosis w audiometry (pt consent given)

Plan: Write to audiologist

Writing Task:

Using the information in the case notes, write a letter of referral to Dr Albury, audiologist, outlining the patient's symptoms, and requesting further investigation and management. Address the letter to Dr Danielle Albury, Audiologist, Newtown Hospital, 123 New Street, Newtown.

In your answer:

- **Expand the relevant notes into complete sentences**
- **Do not use note form**
- **Use letter format**

The body of the letter should be approximately 180–200 words.

Part A

In this part of the test, you'll hear two different extracts. In each extract, a health professional is talking to a patient.

For **questions 1–24**, complete the notes with information you hear.

Now, look at the notes for extract one.

Extract 1: Questions 1–12

You hear a physiotherapist talking to a new patient called Mervin Sprake. For **questions 1–12**, complete the notes with a word or short phrase that you hear.

You now have thirty seconds to look at the notes.

Patient: **Mervyn Sprake**

Background to condition

- experienced (**1**) _____ over a long period
- admits to being both irritable and (**2**) _____ at times
- works as a (**3**) _____
- went through a (**4**) _____ – described as stressful

Onset of symptoms

- unintended weight loss – not accompanied by loss of appetite
- experienced frequent (**5**) _____ (embarrassing)
- hands often felt (**6**) _____ during the working day
- often felt thirsty – led to increased urination
- experienced (**7**) _____ whilst working (took breaks)
- remembers feelings of (**8**) _____ about work and general depression

Diagnosis and treatment

- sought medical help after starting to feel (**9**) '_____' in his movements
- diagnosed with hyperthyroidism
- prescribed carbimazole – had (**10**) _____ as a side effect
- referred to physiotherapy for a (**11**) _____
    n.b. allergy to (**12**) _____

Extract 2: Questions 13–24

You hear a rheumatologist talking to a new patient called Tina Marinov. For questions **13–24**, complete the notes with a word or short phrase that you hear.

You now have thirty seconds to look at the notes.

Patient:	Tina Marinov

Onset of symptoms

- final year university student (geology)

    – generally fit – keen on **(13)** _____ as a leisure pursuit

- long hike on a hot day led to dehydration and episode of

    (14) _____ – attributed to sunstroke

- later noticed facial rash on nose and **(15)** _____ –
  resolved overnight

Development of symptoms

- sudden onset of joint pain – in both knees and **(16)** _____

    – noticeable **(17)** _____ (friends commented)

- sleep affected – followed by day-long **(18)** _____

- diagnosed with flu (fever present) – paracetamol prescribed

- increased sensitivity to cold – pain and discoloration in

    (19) _____

- reports instances of **(20)** _____ and memory issues

- onset of chest pain and **(21)** _____

Investigations and referral

- **(22)** _____ initially suspected (doctor)

- blood test led to diagnosis of **(23)** _____ (family history)

- additional symptom – loss of **(24)** _____ led to referral

- referred for ANA test

Part B

In this part of the test, you'll hear six different extracts. In each extract, you'll hear people talking in a different healthcare setting.

For **questions 25–30**, choose the answer (**A**, **B** or **C**) which fits best according to what you hear. You'll have time to read each question before you listen. Complete your answers as you listen.

Now look at question 25.

Fill the circle in completely. Example: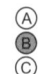

25 You hear a senior practice nurse briefing her team in a local health centre about a new app.

What is she stressing about the app?

Ⓐ Certain patients should be made aware of it.

Ⓑ Patients may need some help in understanding it.

Ⓒ It's intended for healthcare workers rather than patients.

26 You hear a hospital nurse talking to the wife of a patient.

What worries her about his proposed discharge?

Ⓐ dealing with his level of fatigue

Ⓑ how motivated he'll be to keep active

Ⓐ the amount of physical support he'll need

27 You hear a community nurse talking to a patient.

What is the patient concerned about?

(A) the possible recurrence of a condition

(B) discomfort in the site of previous surgery

(C) changes to a growth that's already been examined

28 You hear a discharge nurse talking to a patient who's had minor surgery.

The patient is requesting that a family member

(A) is updated on the next steps in her treatment.

(B) is given the chance to speak to a member of the surgical team.

(C) is allowed to attend a future appointment.

29 You hear two hospital nurses handing over a patient at the change of shift.

What does the incoming nurse agree to do for the patient?

(A) review his analgesia needs

(B) report a possible skin infection

(C) arrange a referral to a specialist

30 You hear the beginning of a training session for healthcare staff in a primary-care setting on the subject of patient consultations.

What is the focus of the session going to be?

(A) alternative ways of setting up consultations

(B) how to make the most of telephone consultations

(C) ways of deciding when face-to-face consultations are necessary

Part C

In this part of the test, you'll hear two different extracts. In each extract, you'll hear health professionals talking about aspects of their work.

For **questions 31–42**, choose the answer (**A**, **B** or **C**) which fits best according to what you hear. Complete your answers as you listen.

Now look at extract one.

Fill the circle in completely. Example:

Extract 1: Questions 31–36

You hear an interview with an occupational therapist called Denise Bronner, who's talking about her work and training.

You now have 90 seconds to read **questions 31–36**.

31 When she was working at an animal-rescue centre, Denise came to realise that

   (A)   the centre's policy towards dog owners was misguided.

   (B)   her idea of reuniting dogs with their owners was unrealistic.

   (C)   some dogs represented a valuable source of support for their owners.

32 What did Denise find particularly rewarding about her job in residential care?

   (A)   the wide range of people she got to work with

   (B)   the holistic nature of the support that she provided

   (C)   the opportunity to use some of her previous experience

33 What does Denise highlight about her Occupational Therapy training?

   (A)   how challenging it was working in such a wide range of environments

   (B)   how effectively theory and practice complemented each other

   (C)   how broad her background reading was required to be

34 The main thing Denise learnt from her placement in an intensive-care unit was

   Ⓐ the value of effective multi-disciplinary teamwork.

   Ⓑ the best way of monitoring each patient's progress.

   Ⓒ the need to adapt her input to the specific setting.

35 What aspect of Denise's placement in the Stroke Unit has since proved most useful to her?

   Ⓐ being given responsibility for her own project

   Ⓑ working with patients from a particular age group

   Ⓒ gaining experience of a key skill in her specialism

36 In the case of the patient called Malcolm, Denise's task was to

   Ⓐ help him find the motivation to make progress.

   Ⓑ convince him to adhere to an exercise programme.

   Ⓒ give him practice in strategies he'd need after his discharge.

Now look at extract two.

Extract 2: Questions 37–42

You hear Dr Karl Bornholm giving a presentation about the diagnosis and treatment of childhood asthma.

You now have 90 seconds to read **questions 37–42**.

37 In his introduction to the topic of childhood asthma, Dr Bornholm expresses his

    (A) frustration at the lack of consistent guidance for doctors.

    (B) regret that more isn't being done to combat the disease.

    (C) surprise that recent findings aren't informing practice.

38 What does Dr Bornholm suggest about the word 'asthma'?

    (A) It should be replaced with a more meaningful term.

    (B) Its use should be restricted to its most general meaning.

    (C) A range of terms should be adopted that modify its meaning.

39 Dr Bornholm feels that failure to accurately diagnose asthma in children can only be addressed by

    (A) identifying the single root cause of the problem worldwide.

    (B) adopting a targeted approach to deal with it in each region.

    (C) accepting there are regional variations in what causes the problem.

40 With regard to children under the age of three, Dr Bornholm points out that

   (A) there's a reluctance to use any form of asthma testing.

   (B) accepted means of testing for asthma would be inappropriate.

   (C) disagreement exists regarding the best form of asthma test to use.

41 Dr Bornholm feels that to address the needs of teenagers with asthma, it's necessary to

   (A) treat patients of each gender differently.

   (B) give them a wider choice of treatment pathways.

   (C) accept that they may not manage their medication reliably.

42 What does Dr Bornholm see as the priority for dealing with childhood asthma?

   (A) the development of a range of tools for monitoring the condition

   (B) further research to identify common triggers in the onset of asthma

   (C) a focus on identifying those aspects of the condition that are treatable

OET SAMPLE TEST

ROLEPLAYER CARD NO. 1	MEDICINE

SETTING   Doctor's Clinic

PATIENT   You are 28 years old and you have a lump in your groin which is causing discomfort. The doctor has just finished examining you.

TASK

- When asked, say you first noticed the lump about three weeks ago. It hasn't changed since then. You can feel a burning, aching sensation in your groin.

- When asked, say you go to the gym every day and lift weights. You're not constipated, you don't have a cough, and you've never had surgery.

- Say you really don't want surgery. You're worried about all the risks and complications that can result from surgery.

- Say you didn't realise a hernia could be life-threatening, so you'll have the surgery as advised.

- Say you'll follow the advice on self-care until you can have surgery.

© Cambridge Boxhill Language Assessment (2022)   SAMPLE TEST

OET SAMPLE TEST

CANDIDATE CARD NO. 1	MEDICINE

SETTING   Doctor's Clinic

DOCTOR   Your patient is 28 years old and has a lump in his/her groin which is causing discomfort. You have just finished examining the patient. You diagnose an indirect inguinal hernia.

TASK

- Find out more details about patient's lump (e.g., onset, progression, pain/discomfort characteristics, etc.).

- Explore patient's risk factors of hernia (e.g., heavy lifting, constipation, prolonged coughing, prior surgery, etc.).

- Give diagnosis of hernia (e.g., intestinal protrusion through abdominal wall weakness, congenital defect, worsened by strenuous activities, etc.). Recommend surgery (e.g., outpatient procedure, typically laparoscopic repair with surgical mesh etc.).

- Reassure patient about hernia surgery (e.g., risks/complications rare, common procedure, etc.). Stress risks of not having surgery (e.g., pressure on surrounding tissue, potential for bowel obstruction/strangulation, possibly life-threatening, etc.).

- Advise patient on self-care while waiting for surgery (e.g., padded belt for support, pain relief as required, no heavy lifting, etc.).

© Cambridge Boxhill Language Assessment (2022)   SAMPLE TEST

OET SAMPLE TEST

ROLEPLAYER CARD NO. 2	MEDICINE

SETTING   Nursing home facility

CARER   Your 89-year-old mother resides in a nursing home facility, where you visit her every day. Your mother is currently being treated for aspiration pneumonia. You have asked to speak to the doctor to find out how your mother is.

TASK
- When asked, say you want the doctor's opinion about how your mother is, and whether or not she's getting any better.
- Say your mother has been on antibiotics for 24 hours, so you thought there would be more improvement by now.
- Say you don't have any specific concerns, but you always worry about your mother and whether she's being looked after properly.
- Say you're glad to hear she's receiving good care. You're going to take her outside for a couple of hours when she wakes up.
- Say you think it will be good for her to have a change of scenery and to get some fresh air.
- Say you hadn't thought about the dangers. You'll wait a few days before taking her outside.

SAMPLE TEST

OET SAMPLE TEST

CANDIDATE CARD NO. 2	MEDICINE

SETTING   Nursing home facility

DOCTOR   This carer has asked to speak to you about his/her 89-year-old mother, who is being treated for aspiration pneumonia. You first met this carer yesterday when you diagnosed his/her mother's illness. The mother is not present during this discussion.

TASK
- Find out reason for carer's request to see you.
- Update carer on his/her mother's progress (e.g., vital signs reassuring, well-hydrated, plenty of restorative sleep, etc.).
- Give information about recovery from aspiration pneumonia (e.g., 48 hours required for treatment effect, coughing expected for 4–6 weeks, possible tiredness/weakness for three months, etc.). Find out if carer has any other concerns.
- Reassure carer about level of mother's care (e.g., constant supervision, physical/pulmonary rehabilitation, positioning for feeding, nutritional support, etc.).
- Advise need for mother to remain in bed (e.g., monitoring required, importance of rest, etc.).
- Warn of risks of taking mother outside (e.g., dehydration, vulnerability to dust/pollen/smoke, etc.). Recommend waiting for a few days (e.g., less frequent monitoring, mother's condition improved/more stable, etc.).

SAMPLE TEST

Writing marking criteria

OET WRITING Assessment Criteria and Level Descriptors

Band	Purpose	Content	Conciseness & Clarity	Genre & Style	Organisation & Layout	Language
7	Purpose of document is immediately apparent and sufficiently expanded as required	Content is appropriate to intended reader and addresses what is needed to continue care (key information is included; no important details missing); content from case notes is accurately represented	Length of document is appropriate to case and reader (no irrelevant information included); information is summarised effectively and presented clearly	Writing is clinical/factual and appropriate to genre and reader (discipline and knowledge); technical language, abbreviations and polite language are used appropriately for document and recipient	Organisation and paragraphing are appropriate, logical and clear; key information is highlighted and sub-sections are well organised; document is well laid out	Language features (spelling/punctuation/vocabulary/grammar/sentence structure) are accurate and do not interfere with meaning
6				Performance shares features of bands 5 and 7		
5	Purpose of document is apparent but not sufficiently highlighted or expanded	Content is appropriate to intended reader and mostly addresses what is needed to continue care; content from case notes is generally accurately represented	Length of document is mostly appropriate to case and reader; information is mostly summarised effectively and presented clearly	Writing is clinical/factual and appropriate to genre and reader with occasional, minor inappropriacies; technical language, abbreviations and polite language are used appropriately with minor inconsistencies	Organisation and paragraphing are generally appropriate, logical and clear; occasional lapses of organisation in sub-sections and/or highlighting of key information; layout is generally good	Minor slips in language generally do not interfere with meaning
4				Performance shares features of bands 3 and 5		
3	Purpose of document is not immediately apparent and may show very limited expansion	Content is mostly appropriate to intended reader; some key information (about case or to continue care) may be missing; there may be some inaccuracies in content	Inclusion of some irrelevant information distracts from overall clarity of document; attempt to summarise only partially successful	Writing is at times inappropriate to the document or target reader; over-reliance on technical language and abbreviations may distract reader	Organisation and paragraphing are not always logical, creating strain for the reader; key information may not be highlighted; layout is mostly appropriate with some lapses	Inaccuracies in language, in particular in complex structures, cause minor strain for the reader but do not interfere with meaning
2				Performance shares features of bands 1 and 3		
1	Purpose of document is partially obscured/unclear and/or misunderstood	Content does not provide intended reader sufficient information about the case and what is needed to continue care; key information is missing or inaccurate	Clarity of document is obscured by the inclusion of many unnecessary details; attempt to summarise not successful	The writing shows inadequate understanding of the genre and target reader; mis- or over-use of technical language and abbreviations cause strain for the reader	Organisation not logical, putting strain on the reader; or heavy reliance on case note structure; key information is not well highlighted and the layout may not be appropriate	Inaccuracies in language cause considerable strain for the reader and may interfere with meaning
0				Performance below Band 1		

© OET – 2019

Writing marking criteria

OET OCCUPATIONAL ENGLISH TEST
WRITING Assessment Criteria and Level Descriptors

Criterion	Description
Purpose • Helps the reader get a **quick and precise sense** of what is asked of them	Due to time constraints, health professionals want to understand the purpose behind a written handover document (e.g. referral letter) very quickly and efficiently. This criterion therefore examines how clearly the writing communicates the purpose of the document to the reader. The purpose for writing should be introduced early in the document and then clearly expanded on later (often near the end of the document). The purpose should be easily and immediately identifiable to the reader, so there is no need to search for it.

Content
• Considers **necessary information** (audience awareness: what does the reader need to know?)
• Considers **accuracy** of information
	The content criterion examines a number of aspects of the content:
	   • All key information is included
	   • Information is accurately represented
	Audience awareness is key here. The writing needs to be appropriate to the reader (and their knowledge of the case) and what they need to know to continue care.

Conciseness & Clarity
• Considers **irrelevant information** (audience awareness: what doesn't the reader need to know?)
• Considers how **effectively** the case is **summarised** (audience awareness: no time is wasted)
	Health professionals value concise and clear communication. This criterion, therefore also considers:
	   • whether unnecessary information from the notes is included and how distracting this may be to the reader, i.e. Does this affect clarity? Is there any information that could be left out?
	   • how well the information (the case) is summarised and how clearly this summary is presented to the reader.

Genre & Style • Considers the **appropriateness** of features such as **register and tone** to the document's purpose and audience	Referral letters and similar written handover documents need to show awareness of genre by being written in a clinical/factual manner (e.g. not including personal feelings and judgements) and awareness of the target reader through using professional register and tone. The use of abbreviations should not be overdone thereby assuming common prior knowledge. If written to a medical colleague in a similar discipline, then judicious use of abbreviations and technical terms would be entirely appropriate, but if the medical colleague was in a totally different discipline, or a letter was from a specialist to a GP, more explanation and less shorthand would be desirable. If the target readership includes the patient, the information must be worded appropriately, e.g. minimising medical jargon.
Organisation & Layout • Considers **organisational features** of the document	Health professionals value documents that are clearly structured so it is easy for them to efficiently retrieve relevant information. This criterion examines how well the document is organised and laid out. It examines whether the paragraphing is appropriate, whether sub-sections within the document are logically organised and whether key information is clearly highlighted to the reader so that it is not easily missed. The criterion also considers whether the layout of the document is appropriate.
Language • Considers aspects of language proficiency such as **vocabulary, grammar, spelling, punctuation**	Health professionals are concerned with linguistic features only to the extent that they facilitate or obstruct retrieval of information. This criterion examines whether the language is accurate, used appropriately and whether it interferes with reading comprehension or speed.

© OET – 2019

Speaking marking criteria

I. Linguistic Criteria

Band	Intelligibility	Fluency	Appropriateness of Language	Resources of Grammar and Expression
6	• Pronunciation is easily understood and prosodic features (stress, intonation, rhythm) are used effectively. • L1 accent has no effect on intelligibility.	• Completely fluent speech at normal speed. • Any hesitation is appropriate and not a sign of searching for words or structures.	• Entirely appropriate register, tone and lexis for the context. • No difficulty at all in explaining technical matters in lay terms.	• Rich and flexible. • Wide range of grammar and vocabulary used accurately and flexibly. • Confident use of idiomatic speech.
5	• Easily understood. • Communication is not impeded by a few pronunciation or prosodic errors and/or noticeable L1 accent. • Minimal strain for the listener.	• Fluent speech at normal speed, with only occasional repetition or self-correction. • Hesitation may occasionally indicate searching for words or structures, but is generally appropriate.	• Mostly appropriate register, tone and lexis for the context. • Occasional lapses are not intrusive.	• Wide range of grammar and vocabulary generally used accurately and flexibly. • Occasional errors in grammar or vocabulary are not intrusive.
4	• Easily understood most of the time. • Pronunciation or prosodic errors and/or L1 accent at times cause strain for the listener.	• Uneven flow, with some repetition, especially in longer utterances. • Some evidence of searching for words, which does not cause serious strain. • Delivery may be staccato or too fast/slow.	• Generally appropriate register, tone and lexis for the context, but somewhat restricted and lacking in complexity. • Lapses are noticeable and at times reflect limited resources of grammar and expression.	• Sufficient resources to maintain the interaction. • Inaccuracies in vocabulary and grammar, particularly in more complex sentences, are sometimes intrusive. • Meaning is generally clear.
3	• Produces some acceptable features of spoken English. • Difficult to understand because errors in pronunciation/stress/intonation and/or L1 accent cause serious strain for the listener.	• Very uneven. • Frequent pauses and repetitions indicate searching for words or structures. • Excessive use of fillers and difficulty sustaining longer utterances cause serious strain for the listener.	• Some evidence of appropriate register, tone and lexis, but lapses are frequent and intrusive, reflecting inadequate resources of grammar and expression.	• Limited vocabulary and control of grammatical structures, except very simple sentences. • Persistent inaccuracies are intrusive.
2	• Often unintelligible. • Frequent errors in pronunciation/stress/intonation and/or L1 accent cause severe strain for the listener.	• Extremely uneven. • Long pauses, numerous repetition and self-corrections make speech difficult to follow.	• Mostly inappropriate register, tone and lexis for the context.	• Very limited resources of vocabulary and grammar, even in simple sentences. • Numerous errors in word choice.
1	• Almost entirely unintelligible.	• Impossible to follow, consisting of isolated words and phrases and self-corrections, separated by long pauses.	• Entirely inappropriate register, tone and lexis for the context.	• Limited in all respects.
0	• Candidate does not provide any response.			

Speaking marking criteria

II. Clinical Communication Criteria

In the role play, there is evidence of the test taker …

A. Indicators of relationship building

A1	initiating the interaction appropriately (greeting, introductions, nature of interview)
A2	demonstrating an attentive and respectful attitude
A3	adopting a non-judgemental approach
A4	showing empathy for feelings/predicament/emotional state

A: Relationship building
- 3 – Adept use
- 2 – Competent use
- 1 – Partially effective use
- 0 – Ineffective use

B. Indicators of understanding & incorporating the patient's perspective

B1	eliciting and exploring the patient's ideas/concerns/expectations
B2	picking up the patient's cues
B3	relating explanations to elicited ideas/concerns/expectations

B. Understanding & incorporating the patient's perspective
- 3 – Adept use
- 2 – Competent use
- 1 – Partially effective use
- 0 – Ineffective use

C. Indicators of providing structure

C1	sequencing the interview purposefully and logically
C2	signposting changes in topic
C3	using organising techniques in explanations

C. Providing structure
- 3 – Adept use
- 2 – Competent use
- 1 – Partially effective use
- 0 – Ineffective use

D. Indicators for information gathering

D1	facilitating the patient's narrative with active listening techniques, minimising interruption
D2	using initially open questions, appropriately moving to closed questions
D3	NOT using compound questions/leading questions
D4	clarifying statements which are vague or need amplification
D5	summarising information to encourage correction/invite further information

D. Information gathering
- 3 – Adept use
- 2 – Competent use
- 1 – Partially effective use
- 0 – Ineffective use

E. Indicators for information giving

E1	establishing initially what the patient already knows
E2	pausing periodically when giving information, using the response to guide next steps
E3	encouraging the patient to contribute reactions/feelings
E4	checking whether the patient has understood information
E5	discovering what further information the patient needs

E. Information giving
- 3 – Adept use
- 2 – Competent use
- 1 – Partially effective use
- 0 – Ineffective use

Writing booklet sample

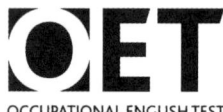

WRITING SUB-TEST – ANSWER BOOKLET

CANDIDATE NUMBER:

LAST NAME:

FIRST NAME:

MIDDLE NAMES:

PROFESSION:

VENUE:

TEST DATE:

Candidate details and photo will be printed here.

Passport Photo

CANDIDATE DECLARATION

By signing this, you agree not to disclose or use in any way (other than to take the test) or assist any other person to disclose or use any OET test or sub-test content. If you cheat or assist in any cheating, use any unfair practice, break any of the rules or regulations, or ignore any advice or information, you may be disqualified and your results may not be issued at the sole discretion of CBLA. CBLA also reserves its right to take further disciplinary action against you and to pursue any other remedies permitted by law. If a candidate is suspected of and investigated for malpractice, their personal details and details of the investigation may be passed to a third party where required.

CANDIDATE SIGNATURE: _____

TIME ALLOWED
READING TIME: 5 MINUTES
WRITING TIME: 40 MINUTES

INSTRUCTIONS TO CANDIDATES

1. **Reading time: 5 minutes**
   During this time you may study the writing task and notes. You **MUST NOT** write, highlight, underline or make any notes.

2. **Writing time: 40 minutes**

3. Use the back page for notes and rough draft only. Notes and rough draft will **NOT** be marked.

   Please write your answer clearly on page 1 and page 2.

   Cross out anything you **DO NOT** want the examiner to consider.

4. You must write your answer for the Writing sub-test in this **Answer Booklet** using **pen or pencil**.

5. You must **NOT** remove OET material from the test room.

www.occupationalenglishtest.org
© Cambridge Boxhill Language Assessment – ABN 51 988 559 414

[CANDIDATE NO.] WRITING SUB-TEST ANSWER BOOKLET 01/04

Photocopiable

Writing booklet sample

Please record your answer on this page.

(Only answers on Page 1 and Page 2 will be marked.)

_____
_____
_____
_____
_____
_____
_____
_____
_____
_____
_____
_____
_____
_____
_____
_____
_____
_____
_____
_____
_____
_____
_____
_____
_____
_____
_____
_____
_____

- - - - - - - - - - DO NOT WRITE ON QR CODE - - - - - - - - - -

DO NOT WRITE ON QR CODE

OET Writing sub-test – Answer booklet   1

[CANDIDATE NO.]   WRITING SUB-TEST - ANSWER BOOKLET 02/04

Writing booklet sample

Please record your answer on this page.

(Only answers on Page 1 and Page 2 will be marked.)

OET Writing sub-test – Answer booklet   2

[CANDIDATE NO.] WRITING SUB-TEST - ANSWER BOOKLET 03/04

Writing booklet sample

Space for notes and rough draft. Only your answers on Page 1 and Page 2 will be marked.